LOW FODMAP RECIPES

The Complete Guide and Cookbook for Beginners

(Health Diet Plan to Beat Bloat and Soothe Your Gut With Recipes)

Lee Pride

Published by Alex Howard

© **Lee Pride**

All Rights Reserved

Low Fodmap Recipes: The Complete Guide and Cookbook for Beginners (Health Diet Plan to Beat Bloat and Soothe Your Gut With Recipes)

ISBN 978-1-990169-21-2

All rights reserved. No part of this guide may be reproduced in any form without permission in writing from the publisher except in the case of brief quotations embodied in critical articles or reviews.

Legal & Disclaimer

The information contained in this book is not designed to replace or take the place of any form of medicine or professional medical advice. The information in this book has been provided for educational and entertainment purposes only.

The information contained in this book has been compiled from sources deemed reliable, and it is accurate to the best of the Author's knowledge; however, the Author cannot guarantee its accuracy and validity and cannot be held liable for any errors or omissions. Changes are periodically made to this book. You must consult your doctor or get professional medical advice before using any of the suggested remedies, techniques, or information in this book.

Table of contents

PART 1 1

INTRODUCTION 2

GASTROINTESTINAL DISORDERS 2
THE FODMAP: WHAT ARE THEY? 3

CHAPTER 1: LOW-FODMAP DIET 6

WHEN YOU CAN START THE LOW DIET FODMAP? 6
THE PHASES OF THE DIET 6
THE EFFECTIVENESS OF THE LOW DIET FODMAP 10
LOW-FODMAP: GENERAL INDICATION 11
THE FOODS TO AVOID 13
PERMITS FOODS 16
WHAT IF THE LOW-FODMAP DOES NOT WORK? 20
THE DIET LOW-FODMAP WHEN YOU DO NOT EAT AT HOME 23
PROBLEMS WITH FOOD NO FODMAP 24

CHAPTER 2: GOOD ADVICE AND GOOD HABITS 25

KNOW THE FOODS 25

CHAPTER 3: BOWEL DISEASES AND DISORDERS 29

OTHER INTESTINAL DISEASES 29
SIDE EFFECTS OF MEDICATIONS AND SUPPLEMENTS 30
THE IBS IS IT? 30
SIBO (SMALL INTESTINAL BACTERIAL OVERGROWTH) 32
FUNCTIONAL GASTROINTESTINAL DISORDERS (FGID) 36
THE BLOATING, ABDOMINAL DISTENSION THE GAS AND INTESTINAL 38

CROHN'S DISEASE 47

THE ULCERATIVE COLITIS 51

CELIAC DISEASE 58

CHAPTER 4: THE LOW-FODMAP DIET COOKBOOK FOR BREAKFAST 65

COCOA PANCAKE 65

BANANA BREAD 66

CARROT CAKE COCONUT PORRIDGE 67

CARROT CAKE COOKIES 68

GREEN SMOOTHIE BOWL WITH CHIA PUDDING 70

DESERT PETALS 71

BUCKWHEAT AND COCONUT GRANOLA 73

CRISPY CHOCOLATE QUINOA BARS 74

PUMPKIN PANCAKES 75

PUMPKIN AND CHOCOLATE CHIP MUFFINS 76

BAKED MILLET PUDDING WITH PINE NUTS 78

OAT PORRIDGE WITH BLUEBERRY COULIS 79

BUCKWHEAT - COCONUT BISCUITS 80

VANILLA MILLET PORRIDGE 81

CHOCOLATEY OVERNIGHT CHIA AND BANANA OATS 82

CHESTNUT PANCAKES WITH RAW COCOA SPREAD 83

COCONUT CRUMBLE WITH STRAWBERRY AND RHUBARB 84

OATMEAL PANCAKE 86

ROLLED OATS, BRAZIL NUTS AND DARK CHOCOLATE COOKIES 87

CARROT CAKE 88

BUCKWHEAT AND BANANA CAKE 89

HOT CHOCOLATE WITH BRAZIL NUTS 91

CHAPTER 5: THE LOW-FODMAP DIET COOKBOOK FOR APPETIZERS AND MAIN MEALS 92

Millet And Chickpeas Falafel 92

Savory Cake With Beets, Pumpkin And Feta 93

Endive Soup 96

Slow Cooked - Beef Stew 98

Quinoa With Vegetables And Lemon Scent 99

The Veggie Tartare With Lemon Juice 101

Omelette With Sweet Potato, Spinach And Feta 102

Brown Rice Spaghetti With Black Cabbage 103

Vegan Lentil Burgers 104

Polenta Wedges With Red Endive 106

Orange And Thyme Chicken 107

Zucchini Crusted With Fillets Of Plaice 108

Millet Croquettes With Zucchini And Basil 109

Oven-Baked Salmon With Dill 110

Beef Burger With Eggplant Bun 112

Vegetable Curry 113

Quinoa And Spinach Croquettes 114

Dukkah-Crusted Cod Fillets 116

Turmeric And Poppy Seeds Chicken And Veggies 117

Zucchini And Bacon Muffin 118

Carrots And Turmeric Velvety Soup 120

CHAPTER 6: THE LOW-FODMAP DIET COOKBOOK FOR SIDE DISHES 122

Parsnip And Turmeric Cous Cous 122

Kale Chips 123

Braised Red Cabbage 124

Italian Mashed Potatoes 125

No-Fried Chips With Thyme-Scented 125

Fennel And Orange Salad 126

CHAPTER 7: THE LOW-FODMAP DIET COOKBOOK FOR SNACK E SMOOTHIE 127

Gianduia Cream 127
Sunflower Crackers With Sun-Dried Tomatoes And Oregano 127
Matcha And Kiwi Smoothie 128

CHAPTER 8: THE LOW-FODMAP DIET COOKBOOK FOR SAUCES AND CONDIMENTS 129

Spinach Pesto 129
Basil Pesto 130
Winter Pesto 130
Vanilla Dark Chocolate Spread 131
Raspberry Jam And Chia Seeds 132
Yogurt With Tahini 133

CHAPTER 9: THE LOW-FODMAP DIET COOKBOOK FOR DESSERTS 134

Macadamia Nuts Cheesecake With Blueberries 134
Vegan Chocolate Tart 136
Pumpkin And Chocolate Cake 138
Chocolate Truffles 139
Walnuts And Banana Brownie 140
Buckwheat And Banana Cake 141
Strawberry Clafoutis 142

PART 2 144

Anti-Inflammatory Turmeric Shake 172
Cinnamon Hot Chocolate 173
Breads And Breakfast Options 173
Quinoa Protein Porridge 175

Butternut Squash / Pumpkin And Cinnamon Granola	176
Bacon, Sundried Tomato And Courgette Frittata	177
Eggs Muffin Cups Wrapped In Prosciutto	179
Breakfast Burritos	180
Sundried Tomato And Olive Muffins	181
Paleo Focaccia Bread	183
Chocolate Banana Paleo Bread	184
Herb Blinis With Hot Smoked Salmon And Aioli	185
Soups	187
Creamy Carrot Ginger Soup	187
Roasted Red Pepper And Tomato Soup	188

Part 1

Introduction

f you suffer from bloating in the stomach, abdominal pain, and if you have a feeling of fullness in the stomach, try following our LOW-FODMAP method for a couple of weeks. You will learn to know and recognize what you eat. From the knowledge of the results: you'll know which foods to avoid for your specific ailment and the ones that your body can tolerate. Anything you can do it while enjoying our delicious recipes.

The LOW-FODMAP diet is a valuable tool to help those individuals afflicted with recurrent gastrointestinal disorders, of which we were unable to identify a specific trigger, and as such, its use must be followed and evaluated extensively and detailed.

We should not consider it a fad diet but to a path of knowledge, or rather a method that should be used after talking with your doctor and after exams that they may deem necessary.

Thus, a diet can be explored for those who often suffer from bloating, abdominal pain, irregular bowel and has not been able to identify a precise cause for such problems.

Gastrointestinal Disorders

It is estimated that about 22% of the world's population suffers from numerous and troublesome gastrointestinal disorders. Among these disorders are the most common stomach bloating, feelings of fullness, diffuse abdominal pain, flatulence, or diarrhea alternating with constipation. In the presence of these symptoms, it is likely that the cause is Irritable Bowel Syndrome (IBS) or Functional Gastrointestinal Disorders (FGID).

It is idiopathic diseases, which do not have a cause that determines their appearance, for which there are no specific therapies. A suitable system would reduce these nuisances, and disturbances is definitely the one indicated by the LOW-FODMAP diet.

The LOW-FODMAP diet was born in Australia, proposed and tested at the University of Melbourne. In recent years, its use has been the subject of numerous studies that have confirmed good efficacy in reducing symptoms associated with IBS and FGID.

It is a food plan based on the theory that foods containing fermented products, lactose and fructose, alcohol and sugars in general, they would be responsible for certain diseases in the digestive system and of the intestine.

The Fodmap: What Are They?

FODMAP stands for Fermentable-Oligosaccharides-Disaccharides-Monosaccharides-And-Polyols.

These are substances that have three characteristics in common:

- They are poorly absorbed in the small intestine;
- are small molecules that in their chemical structure, recall a lot of water inside the intestine causing diarrhea often;
- They are rapidly metabolized by the intestinal bacterial flora, encouraging a proliferation of the same. This implies a

greater production of intestinal gas with the consequent swelling and abdominal bloating.

Fermentable: It means that they are fermented by bacteria in the large intestine.

Oligosaccharides: That is a few sugars, these molecules are composed of individual sugars joined in a chain (fructans and galactans).

Disaccharides: Double sugar molecule (sucrose and lactose).

Monosaccharides: Single molecule of sugar (fructose).

And

Polyols: Hydrogenated carbohydrates are used as sweeteners to replace sugar.

The properties of these substances, especially in the case of Polyols, which are often used as low-calorie sweeteners in many foods, are now recognized. In fact, on the labels of the products, the risk of laxative effects must be indicated connected as a result of high consumption. The Polyolis are sugars such as sorbitol, mannitol and xylitol, which are poorly absorbed in the small intestine and are subject to fermentation processes that depend on the amount of consumed dose. Sorbitol abounds in rich fructose fruits while the mannitol is found mainly in mushrooms.

Fructose is present in the food is free, it is linked to the glucose forming the sucrose, which is the common table sugar. The absorption is, in fact, better when there is glucose and varies significantly from subject to subject. It is abundant in honey and many fruits. As syrup is widely used in industrial food production (soft drinks, sweets, bakery products).

The fructans are small polymers of fructose found in grains, fruit banana) and in many vegetables: onion, garlic, artichokes. Our intestine does not have the enzymes for the digestion of these compounds, thus forming a substrate creating processes of fermentation by bacteria.

Lactose is a disaccharide found in the milk of all mammals. His digestion depends on an enzyme which, however, is lost during growth. Only a percentage of adults, very different depending on the geographic area, maintains the enzyme and thus the ability to digest this sugar into adulthood. The lactose malabsorption is easily identified with a simple test, a breath test.

The galactans are lactose polymers. They are very abundant in legumes, and in many foods' cornerstone of vegetarian and vegan diets. They are popular in ethnic food, like cabbage and Brussel sprouts.

Chapter 1: low-fodmap diet

When You Can Start The Low Diet Fodmap?

The LOW-FODMAP diet is right for you if:

- You have excess intestinal gas problems, bloating, abdominal pain, diarrhea or constipation;
- You are not able to alleviate these symptoms by changing your style of food and non-food life (drinking more fluids, doing exercise, eating foods with an increased amount of dietary fiber, stress management, sleep better);
- Together with your doctor you have eliminated any possible causes of irritable bowel syndrome that might be the cause of your symptoms and if your doctor has advised you to follow FODMAP method to eliminate the symptoms caused by irritable bowel syndrome.

The Phases Of The Diet

Reduce your intake of foods rich FODMAP, with a diet low content of these substances, is a valuable aid in the treatment of symptoms associated with the 'IBS. The diet consists:

- of a terminal phase, during which they are eliminated from the diet foods richest in FODMAP.
- At the end follows a phase of reintroduction with which are tested foods deleted in the previous step, in order to understand the quantity and frequency of consumption that the subject is able to tolerate.

- The first phase of the LOW-FODMAP diet, therefore, consists of 'total elimination of high FODMAP content foods, the duration of which can vary from two to six weeks, depending on the severity of the symptoms and should be agreed with the gastroenterologist.
- In this period you'll want to create a food diary where you go to record, day by day, meal by meal, all the food consumed.
- This will make it possible, from week to week, reintroducing certain foods, in the reintegration phase, by monitoring their effect and removing them again if the symptoms reappear
- Depending on the individual tolerance, in fact, it may well start to gradually reintroduce the disaccharides such as lactose, then the fruit containing polyols, even after the vegetables and finally the gluten.
- Given the complexity of both procedural and nutrition, we reiterate once again the need to resort to a nutritionist, to reintroduce in the appropriate manner the initially banned foods.

The objective of the first stage is to determine the regression of the symptoms while the purpose of the second phase is to find the proper balance between a good control of symptoms and a more varied diet. In fact, in the elimination phase, we exclude many common foods, causing not only a more complicated power management inside and outside the home but in the long run also possible nutritional deficiencies (such as calcium and iron). In addition, some FODMAP encourages the growth of "good bacteria" in the gut. Thus their very prolonged elimination could have adverse effects in a long time. Once you completed the phase of reintroduction, it will identify those foods responsible for triggering symptoms. This leads to a dietary regime, applicable in the long term. It is a good compromise between power supply more varied and an optimal control of symptoms. Also, it is easier to manage eating out and reintroducing some types of FODMAP, improves the composition of the intestinal bacterial flora.

You can start the re-introduction phase only after reaching a situation of well-being by excluding high FODMAP foods. The degree of improvement in symptoms is variable from person to person, so it is good to establish, together with the Gastroenterologist reference, which is the level of control of symptoms from which one starts.

During the re-introduction, it is essential to keep following the diet LOW-FODMAP and test just one food at a time. Each food must be tested for three consecutive days, in increasing quantities. Quantity is very important because it is related to the onset of symptoms, or certain foods are tolerated only in small amounts. Then it is good to go for 2-3 days before testing another food to prevent the Crusaders effects.

Practical elimination and Reintegration Example

- Have a symptom control for at least three days;
- Consuming a teaspoon of honey a day for three days, always following scrupulously the LOW-FODMAP diet;
- Write down the food diary any symptoms, physical activity, and the most significant emotions;

- Proceed according to the symptoms: if they worsen considerably stop the test immediately, even if they are not spent 3 days. If the symptoms are mild and do not appear, on the third day you may increase the dose to two teaspoons of honey a day and monitor its effects after 1-2 days;
- Once the test with honey, pass 2-3 days following the LOW diet FODMAP, before you begin to try and test another food.

How to read the results:

- If the tested food does not cause any reaction means that it is well tolerated and, once the re-introduction phase, it can be inserted freely in the daily diet.
- If food causes severe symptoms, it is good to interrupt the test and avoid the food in the long term for optimal symptom control.
- If the food causes mild symptoms then it may be retested in smaller doses and less frequent, in order to assess whether a child consumption is well tolerated.

It is not an easy task to interpret all the data collected, so you may want to deal regularly with your gastroenterologist, to avoid unnecessary exclusion of certain foods.

PRACTICAL ADVICE

- You should test foods on days when there is the possibility to have meals at home, or to assign the preparation of someone who is aware of the route taken.
- It is good to maintain a constant and limited consumption of coffee and alcohol throughout the reintroduction phase, since they are substances that can irritate the bowel and a

variable their consumption could interfere with the interpretation of the symptoms.

The Effectiveness Of The Low Diet Fodmap

By learning to know the characteristics of FODMAP, the foods in which they are contained in excessive amounts, how to avoid them and how to gradually reintegrate into our power, we will begin to have a greater understanding of our problems and their causes. Thanks to this method, we will have a resolution of symptoms and improvement in gastrointestinal health. Generally, study the therapeutic efficacy of a diet is not very simple, both for the complexity that many diets often impose on rigid diets that are difficult to follow scrupulously; both because they require substantial changes to the lifestyle of the participants.

One potential problem in LOW-FODMAP diets is the lack of accurate data on the content of these substances in different foods. In addition, there is a difficulty in establishing the of each food consumption threshold values as it is not the content of a single food but the total FODMAP content consumed in the meal to determine the appearance or not of the symptoms.

Before you start a job like this, it would be good to talk with your doctor and possibly run the breath test at least for fructose, lactose and sorbitol to evaluate a possible malabsorption of these sugars.

The LOW-FODMAP diet is not the treatment of Irritable Bowel Syndrome: it is a diet whose aim is to reduce symptoms associated with certain pathologies. The use of diet indicated by the LOW-FODMAP has shown good efficacy and excellent results. Over 70% of the subjects that followed showed great improvements and, after the step of reintroduction of FODMAP, often allows to raise the threshold of tolerance towards trigger foods.

The benefits

The LOW-FODMAP diet, therefore, limiting the consumption of specific foods, is able to ensure a rapid improvement of the symptoms.

Already after a few weeks of dieting:

- It will feel a strong sense of lightness bowel;
- They will reduce the abdominal pain and the strange feeling of unease;
- Improve the acts evacuators, both for consistency for that frequency.

Low-Fodmap: General Indication

The LOW-FODMAP diet is a complex diet. As recalled, initially, you will need to eliminate from your diet all the foods rich in these substances (The FODMAP) for a period ranging from two to six weeks. But, before suggesting a diet of this type, the awareness and the will to start an in-depth individual dietary survey is required in order to understand which foods cause symptoms in each subject. In fact, each subject must have clear dynamics with which certain foods may cause problems and disorders, such as analyzing the frequency of consumption and the total amount of consumed FODMAP is important in determining the accused disorders.

Here are some basic guidelines for good adherence to the diet:

- choose foods in which glucose is more abundant than fructose;
- however, limit the overall consumption of fructose;
- reduce the fructans and galactans consumption;
- if you have tested positive for the breath test for lactose reduce the lactose-rich foods consumption;
- avoid the consumption of polyols, reducing the consumption of foods with sweeteners and fruits such as plums, peaches, plums;
- avoid the consumption of foods mentioned in the following chapter.

If in the course of the diet there was a noise reduction, after a period ranging from two to six weeks, you will start in a carefully re-checked various FODMAP rich foods: the purpose is to determine which foods, such as quantities and with what frequency of consumption, are able to trigger symptoms. Obviously, foods so identified will be consumed very carefully and in measured quantities.

It's important emphasize that a significant role in the development of disorders might also be due to alterations of the intestinal bacterial flora with reduction of species of Bifidobacterium and Lactobacillus, and an increase of Clostriudium, which ferment the FODMAP and they do grow the intestinal bacterial flora small intestine, causing a slowing of intestinal transit. In some cases, it is possible to suggest consumption of probiotics selected in order to correct these imbalances in the intestinal bacterial population.

It's important that the diet plan maintains adequate fiber and starch, to avoid excessive reduction of probiotic material and potential problems with motility, especially in the large intestine, and the potential genesis of cancerous lesions.

It's important not to forget that this is still a diet and like all diets that you intend to follow, which cannot be improvised and must be followed as directed by a familiar professional and practice with this type of diet, in to provide detailed information on the subject foods to avoid completely, on those to be consumed with care and on those that it is possible to consume freely. You must, in fact, be careful not to exclude certain foods without them even have a real need. At the same time, since it is the total content of FODMAP to create problems, you should carefully plan the consumption of certain foods and, if the results were not what we expected,

The Foods To Avoid

always Reiterating the need for professional supervision of nutrition, if I wanted to follow the diet LOW-FODMAP you will need to exercise caution in the consumption of these foods.

Following is a list of high FODMAP foods, even in small portions.

FRUIT

- apricots
- Watermelon

- Avocado
- persimmon
- cherries
- Dates
- figs
- dried fruit
- Mango
- apples
- Blackberries
- peaches
- Pere
- Fresh plums and prunes
- Cashew nuts
- Pistachios

VEGETABLES

- Garlic
- Asparagus
- red beets
- Artichokes
- Cabbages
- Cauliflower
- All types of onions
- mushrooms

CEREALS

- Cereal made with wheat, barley and rye
- Barley
- Wheat products and Kamut as biscuits, flour and pasta
- Rye products like biscuits, flour and bread

DESSERTS

- Molasses
- Honey
- Agave syrup

LEGUMES

- dried chickpeas
- Fresh Beans sechi
- Fava beans
- dried lentils
- dried peas

DAIRY PRODUCT

- Soft cheeses such as mascarpone, ricotta, cream cheese, cottage cheese
- Ice cream
- Kefir
- Condensed milk
- Milk cow, sheep and goat
- Milk powder
- Soy products such as milk and yogurt

DRINKS

- Alcoholic beverages
- Cider
- Fruit juices
- Coffee substitutes
- Vermouth and sweet wines

  MEAT, FISH AND EGGS
- In dishes prepared with high FODMAP contained ingredients such as soup, sauces and sausages.

  Sweeteners OF ANY NATURE.

Permits Foods

Following is a list of foods that have a low content FODMAP and accounted for.

FRUIT

- Citrus fruits (80 g)
- Pineapple (140 g)
- Banana not too mature (100 g)
- Strawberries (150 g)
- Raspberries (60 g)
- Blueberries (40 g)
- Kiwi (maximum 2)
- Litchi (maximum 3)
- Maracuja (maximum 2)
- Honeydew Melon (120 g)
- Coconut (65 g)

- Papaya (140 g)
- Grape (150 g)

  VEGETABLES and HERBS
- Beets (75 g)
- Bok choy (75 g)
- Carrots (up to satiety)
- Chinese cabbage (75 g)
- Red cabbage (75 g)
- Savoy cabbage (40 g)
- Cucumbers (up to satiety)
- Palm hearts (up to satiety)
- Herbs of all kinds
- Green beans (75 g)
- Fennel (45 g)
- Bamboo shoots (75 g)
- Lettuce of all types (up to satiety)
- Mais (middle ear)
- Eggplants (75 g)
- Potatoes (up to satiety)
- Red peppers (to fill)
- Tomatoes (except cherry tomatoes)
- Rape (75 g)
- Radishes (to fill)
- Celery (10 g)

- Celeriac (75 g)
- Spinach (up to satiety)
- Ginger
- Zucchini (65 g)

DRESSING AND FATS

- Vinegar
- Butter
- Tomato paste (only if 100% tomato)
- Ketchup
- mayonnaise
- Margarine
- Oil (all kinds)
- Soy sauce
- Mustard
- various spices

DAIRY AND SUBSTITUTES

- Hemp Drinks (12 cl), almonds (25 cl), rice (20 cl)
- Cheese brie, camembert, cheddar, feta cheese, Gruyere cheese, pecorino (40 g)
- Goat cheese (40 g)
- Milk, yogurt and lactose-free ice cream
- Yogurt coconut (125 g)

DESSERTS

- Dark chocolate (30 g)

- Maple syrup (2 small spoons)
- Rice syrup (1 small spoon)
- whole cane sugar

DRINKS

- water
- Coconut water
- Beer (40 cl)
- Coffee in moderation
- Tea (excluding cha and oolong)
- Herbal teas (except chamomile, fennel and dandelion)
- Wine (maximum 15 cl, always excluded sweet wines and liqueur)

CEREALS

- Amaranth flour
- oatmeal
- Buckwheat
- corn flour
- Mile
- Quinoa
- Rice (except wild rice)
- Sorghum

FOODS RICH IN PROTEIN

- walnuts
- peanuts

- Peanut butter
- Almond Butter
- Hazelnuts
- Pine nuts
- Hemp seeds
- Chia seeds
- Sunflower seeds
- Flax seed
- Sesame seeds
- Pumpkin seeds
- Meat and Poultry (unprocessed)
- Chick peas and lentils in a well-rinsed box (40 g)
- Fish and seafood (not processed)
- eggs

What If The Low-Fodmap Does Not Work?

There are many factors that could cause a meager results of a diet FODMAP or the symptoms remain, as always annoying. Professional and patient must work together and identify what, if any of these factors are at work.

In some cases, when there was a low adherence to the diet, or frequent consumption of meals outside the home, or even the choice of foods that contain illegal ingredients, the operation is relatively easy because a greater attention in the choice of foods to ensure a significant reduction in intake of these small, annoying, and widespread molecules. This way, you can see if you are really in front of one of those subjects that do not respond to diet or persistence of symptoms is due to an approximate and insufficient elimination, the use of drugs or the presence of other foods can cause problems. A well-filled food diary can be a tremendous help.

In cases where they remain relevant alterations of intestinal transit are possible interventions:

- In case of constipation it is possible for example to use small amounts of foods rich in sorbitol and / or fructose, which have an appreciable FODMAP laxative action. In this case, the consumption of modest portions apricot, avocado, mango, apples or pears, might help.
- In subjects in which remains a persistent diarrhea may be worth considering an exclusion even more rigorous than those foods that contain fructose and polyols, combined perhaps targeted use of fibers like psyllium that, with their ability to form gels, can improve stool consistency.
- In some cases it may be appropriate to the use of prebiotics or probiotics targeted, which could help improve the condition of the intestinal microbiota that often these patients present altered. The choice of products to be used depends on the nature of the symptoms reported by the patient and it is important that the use of these supplements can actually help reduce waste hassles.

Not all patients respond well to a LOW-FODMAP diet. The data indicate that a variable percentage between 20 and 30% of the subjects does not present a considerable reduction of IBS symptoms; before abandoning the diet, it is therefore necessary to evaluate whether there are situations that have reduced the effectiveness and whether it is possible to put in place strategies to improve patient response. Always consult with your doctor!

The first thing to check, perhaps with the help of the food diary, it's what the signs in the elimination phase are followed. The LOW-FODMAP is a restrictive diet and not easy to be observed, especially in special situations:

- when the patient consumes a large quantity of packaged products that may contain ingredients with a high content FODMAP not easy to identify. This can be done with many of bakery products devoid of widely used gluten to avoid the consumption of fructans rich cereals: these products may contain inulin appreciable quantities, chicory roots, agave juice, apple / pear juice, fructose, xylitol, sorbitol and other polyols, and thus contribute in a decisive manner to the persistence of the symptoms;
- when the patient consumes few meals with generous portions that can lead to a high load FODMAP;
- when the patient does not cook and does not control the ingredients used in the kitchen and is not adequately supported by family members;
- when the patient is highly sensitive to FODMAP and requires a great deal of attention in eliminating specific foods and portion control than it consumes.

Identifying situations of this type may allow better adherence to diet and then assess whether, with most attention, it should be noted if there is an appreciable reduction in symptoms.

If the LOW-FODMAP diet does not work, you can follow the strategies, attention and possible remedies to reduce IBS symptoms; in particular, get used to a careful reading of labels can afford to avoid the consumption of foods that contain FODMAP rich ingredients, not always easy or immediate identification.

The Diet Low-Fodmap When You Do Not Eat At Home

It can often happen for business or pleasure. Many people may eat more or less frequently outside the home. In these situations, it is difficult to have complete control over the ingredients of the food consumed. Onion and garlic can be present in appreciable amounts in a large number of dishes, and the same can be done with other FODMAP rich foods, not always easy to identify. The risk is even higher if you are traveling and you consume ethnic dishes that can be extremely rich in legumes, cereals, vegetables and other products rich FODMAP very little but still recognizable by the special preparations they undergo.

Unfortunately, unlike what happens with gluten and lactose, we are not yet certified foods LOW- FODMAP and there are no precise rules for the preparation of LOW-FODMAP dishes, so you must be very careful in the selection of food ordered from the restaurant, preferring simple recipes with few ingredients, it is familiar with the contents of the pesky sugars.

Better to be overly cautious than end up consuming large quantities of FOMAP, reducing the effectiveness of the diet appreciably.

Problems With Food No Fodmap

In some individuals who suffer from irritable bowel syndrome symptoms may also be due to other foods, can cause bothersome symptoms through entirely different mechanisms:

- In susceptible individuals a high fat intake can cause dyspepsia, abdominal pain, bloating, flatulence and poorly formed stools;
- Coffee can cause diarrhea: caffeine stimulates the motor activity of the colon and may result in dyspepsia and abdominal pain;
- Alcohol can cause digestive problems, nausea, and diarrhea;
- Excessive use of certain types of fibers, such as inulin and wheat bran or oats, may produce bloating and abdominal pain.
- Remarkably, before facing a FODMAP diet it would be appropriate to assess whether the patient presents intolerance to gluten and lactose or other less common intolerances - histamine and amines endogenous, sulfites, salicylates, in order to exclude potential disturbances despite careful elimination.

Chapter 2: good advice and good habits

Know The Foods

Eat a varied and balanced diet

- FLESH: white and red meat, preferring the lean parts can be eaten. Avoid fatty meats such as hot dogs, sausages, bacon, game. Frequency of consumption: 1 red meat once a week, white meat 3-4 times.
- FISH: prefer lean fish (cod, sole, hake, dogfish, trout, sea bream, sea bass, plaice) or fresh oily fish (sardines, mackerel, anchovies), avoid shellfish. The frequency of consumption is at least 2-3 times a week.
- CHEESE: limit consumption to 1-2 times per week, avoiding those seasoned / blue cheeses (pecorino, Gorgonzola, Taleggio), and preferring fresh ones lactose (ricotta, mozzarella).
- EGGS: consume up 1-2 eggs a week, preferably not fried.
- THIN SLICED: raw or cooked ham (lactose) degreased, dried beef, turkey breast, bacon fat. Avoid other meats or sausages. Frequency: 1-2 times a week.
- MILK AND YOGURT WITHOUT LACTOSE: 1-2 servings a day are recommended (eg: 1 glass of milk at breakfast and 1 low-fat yogurt as a snack).

- FRUIT AND VEGETABLES: prefer those to the season, in the permitted quality. Fruit: 2-3 servings per day, for up to 240g. Vegetables: 1 serving lunch and one dinner portion
- GRAIN AND DERIVATIVES: means bread, pasta and bakery products (crackers, breadsticks, biscuits) based on the permitted flour, rice, potatoes, polenta. It is important that they are present 1-2 portions to all the main meals. It is advisable to avoid the whole variety (eg, brown rice), except in case of persistent constipation. Avoid consumption of pizza.
- SWEET: an excess of sugar can increase symptoms, so it is best to limit the intake of sweets (cakes, ice cream, chocolate, jam, cream, puddings, packaged snacks, sweets).
- EXTRA VIRGIN OLIVE OIL (Ages): extra virgin olive oil is to be preferred as a condiment, while it is good to avoid butter, margarine, lard and cream. It is preferable to use the oil raw, average amount of 3-4 tablespoons a day. You can season with herbs, lemon juice, vinegar. Avoid garlic.
- PHYSICAL ACTIVITY: physical activity can be of great help for those suffering from IBS. Exercise helps reduce stress levels and improve symptoms. Not only does physical activity help us achieve and maintain an ideal body weight, but it also helps prevent many diseases (high cholesterol, diabetes, high blood pressure, heart disease).
- It would be good to do 30 minutes a day of exercise. Aerobic activities such as swimming, walking, cycling and dancing should be preferred. Even "invisible" physical activity can

help, that is, the activities we carry out every day (climbing stairs, walking, ...).
- It is suggested to divide the daily nutrition in 3 main meals and 1-2 snacks. It should carve out the right time to dine in peace, chewing long.
- WATER: it is important to hydrate properly during the day. It would be good to drink 1.5-2 liters of water a day, not too cold. You can also introduce liquid form of the decaffeinated tea, herbal tea or chamomile, taking care to avoid the peach tea or tisane of fruits unfit.
- Consume in moderation: tea, coffee (up to 1-2 cups a day), red or white wine (up to 1-2 glasses a day, preferably with meals), juice or orange juice.
- They are to avoid soft drinks, beer, spirits, barley coffee and chicory.
- The carbonated water is instead a good digestive aid.
- Use healthy cooking methods without using fats: Steaming, grilled, roasted, baked, in non-stick pans. It is recommended to avoid fries and not to accompany the dishes with sauces or elaborate sauces (mayonnaise, ketchup, mustard, mustard).
- FOOD LABELS: packaged products can hide FODMAP and therefore it is important to carefully read the list of ingredients on the label.
- GLUTEN FREE PRODUCTS: free diet FODMAP not correspond to follow a gluten-free diet, although the gluten-free

products represent a viable alternative to cereal to exclude. Not all gluten-free products are less incapable!

- Candy and chewing gum, sugarless sweeteners are often sweetened with not allowed.
- Some baked goods may be enriched with INULIN, a vegetable fiber derived from chicory, with a high FODMAP content.
- Often fructose it is added in jams, yoghurts and cereals for breakfast.
- The meat, as well as fish and eggs, is a food without the FODMAP.
- Attention should be given to meat and processed fish (hamburgers, meatballs, breaded fish) and egg (cream products, puddings, sauces) that could contain illegal ingredients.

The Mediterranean diet is a healthy diet pattern for all.

Chapter 3: bowel diseases and disorders

Other Intestinal Diseases

Many of the typical symptoms of certain inflammatory bowel diseases such as Crohn's disease and ulcerative colitis are similar to those of irritable bowel syndrome. For this reason, before starting LOW-FODMAP diet it is good to understand if the symptoms can't be reported due to these diseases: characteristic features are the presence of blood in the stool, anemia, weight loss, persistent fever.

The same considerations apply for the possible presence of a celiac disease. Patients who suffer from this condition often have many of the typical symptoms of IBS and LOW-FODMAP diet that eliminates gluten-containing grains, may delay diagnosis of a disease that can give very serious complications. Here are some typical signs that must be carefully considered: weight loss, iron deficiency, albumin and calcium, iron deficiency anemia, dermatitis, thyroid disease and type 1 diabetes, the latter particularly in children.

The FODMAP diet used blindly can be dangerous and should always be preceded by a careful history and tests that the doctor feels necessary, to avoid masking more serious diseases that in addition to dietary intervention may require and benefit significantly from pharmacological therapy.

For the reasons given and to provide our readers with a comprehensive argumentation and knowledge on the subject, we will analyze the most common intestinal diseases.

Side Effects Of Medications And Supplements

Some medications and supplements can have of the bowel side effects. Their continued use could then contribute to the persistence of specific symptoms:

- The use of antibiotics can cause diarrhea and gastric disorders;
- Codeine, found in many pain relievers, may cause constipation;
- The iron, often found in many supplements can cause constipation;
- Magnesium, often integrated mineral else, it can cause nausea, bloating and diarrhea;
- Metformin, used in the treatment of type 2 diabetes, can cause nausea, abdominal pain and diarrhea.

The Ibs Is It?

Irritable Bowel Syndrome (IBS), is a condition that manifests itself with varying intensity across multiple symptoms which include abdominal pain and discomfort associated with diarrhea and / or constipation or both alternating disorders.

The symptoms are different from person to person, in some cases they can also greatly affect the quality of life.

This problem, long identified with the term colitis or irritable bowel syndrome, is more precisely defined today Irritable Bowel

Syndrome (IBS) to indicate an interest of not only the colon but the entire intestine.

IBS is very common in the population and is more common in women.

Typical symptoms are often identifiable in cramping pain and in altering the characteristics of evacuation of stool and frequency (three times a day to three times a week). Even the need for evacuation effort, feeling of incomplete emptying, the presence of mucus in the stool, and worsening after meals, contribute to the exacerbation of pain.

The IBS is a chronic disorder that alternates periods of aggravation in remission phases and is divided, depending on the most common disorders, in:

IBS-C (C: constipation): IBS characterized by the presence of constipation. More common in women.

- IBS-D (D: diarrhea): IBS characterized by the presence of diarrhea. More common in men.
- IBS-A (A: alternating): IBS alternating periods of constipation and diarrhea periods.

The exact causes that lead to the IBS are not yet fully known. The opinion shared by the experts is that it is a multifactorial disorder where many factors can influence the onset of symptoms, including psychological factors are not negligible such as anxiety, stress and nervousness.

Beyond the variability of symptoms resulting from different causes, it is important to understand that IBS symptoms are partly due to an increased permeability of the intestinal mucosa, which exposes the underlying layers to a non-physiological contact with irritant substances normally present in 'intestines, making it hypersensitive.

Sibo (Small Intestinal Bacterial Overgrowth)

SIBO is a still poorly understood pathological condition of interest in gastroenterology, defined as a syndrome Over-Bacterial growth of the small intestine, or the first part of the intestine, the one adjacent to the stomach and destined to the absorption of most nutrients.

In particular, it assists both to a high growth of the bacterial population in a seat usually less populated, with a concentration of bacteria duodenal greater than 105 CFU / ml, both to a shift in the natural ecosystem intestinal balance with abnormal abuse of certain bacterial species , in particular anaerobic.

While the bacteria are an essential part of a healthy intestine and the large intestine will play important functions, bacterial growth (or the wrong type of microorganisms) in the small intestine may lead to intestinal permeability and a host of other symptoms also very debilitating.

The role of the small intestine in our bodies is very important. Its main function is to help us digest and absorb nutrients from food. It also has an important function for our immune system that contains a large number of lymphoid cells (help us fight infections and others).

The bacteria in its interior, which are less than 1/1000 of those present in the large intestine, help to protect us from pathogenic microorganisms and yeasts that ingest.

At a certain point, however, something happens that breaks this healthy balance of the small intestine, which leads to increase the number of bacteria or bears at its inner different types that normally should not be found there, because migrate from the colon.

To explain in a few words what SIBO simply this sentence: is a colon from the small intestine bacterial migration (or overgrowth) that breaks the natural balance in our intestines and therefore creates a range of annoying and important symptoms.

Symptoms

The symptoms are common to many other diseases, so the recognition of this condition is not always straightforward: diarrhea, abdominal swelling, bloating and chronic abdominal pain may be symptoms related to SIBO, but must exclude many other possible problems, from gastritis syndrome the irritable bowel syndrome, allergies and intolerances. Mild cases are often characterized by alternating constipation and diarrhea, and in the most severe forms (fortunately rare) may also appear malabsorption of vitamin B12 and anemia.

Diagnosis

To diagnose just a simple and painless examination, which is the breath test to lactulose (not to be confused with the Breath Test to lactose which is used to diagnose a possible lactose intolerance). The Breath Test to Lactulose is an absolutely non-invasive test which consists in making exhale patients in a bag for the first time before the intake of lactulose, or a synthetic sugar, and then every 15 minutes during 4 hours thereafter. A sophisticated dedicated equipment then analyzes the composition of breathing in order to detect the amount of expired air before and after taking lactulose.

The fermentation of lactulose by intestinal bacteria, in fact, causes, after a certain time after its ingestion, an increase in the hydrogen content of exhaled air. The lactulose is able to arrive intact at the level of the colon, where the bacterial flora is, however, able to metabolize leading to the production of hydrogen which, consequently, will appear in the patient's breath. The normal time of occurrence of the peak in the breath hydrogen is between 30 and 90 minutes. lower or higher time may indicate the presence of conditions that hinder the normal intestinal transit. The test takes about 4 hours. To run properly, it is important so that the patient adheres to a few pointers that will be indicated when booking.

Dieting LOW-FODMAP and SIBO

Once the pathological condition is detected, a complementary approach is useful in addition to the pharmacological therapy indicated by the attending physician. This involves the use of probiotics, phytotherapy and proper nutrition, which plays an important role in preventing and maintaining a healthy state of our intestines. A diet low in simple and fermentable sugars (FODMAP) can be useful.

Causes

There are some predisposing factors for SIBO but there may also be resulting symptoms of this syndrome. Unfortunately, in this condition, it always creates a vicious circle.

Among the predisposing factors include:

- hypochlorhydria - It is a condition where the acid in the stomach is insufficient to properly digest the proteins and this prevents to absorb the necessary nutrients and it causes putrefaction or fermentation giving rise to inflammation, in production of gas (hydrogen) and ammonia. Since one of the main defense mechanisms that prevent It will also establish the SIBO there is adequate pancreatic and gastric acid secretion, in addition to immune issues and normal intestinal motility, the most frequent cause has been traced to the continuous therapy with proton pump inhibitors (PPI), or more familiarly known as "stomach protectors". These drugs, in fact, not only by reducing the acidity of gastric contents, but also of the environment in the first tract of the intestine, can promote uncontrolled proliferation of certain pathogenic bacterial species. Other times SIBO may be secondary to interventions in the stomach or intestine, in conditions of celiac disease or lactose intolerance not recognized and treated or other medical therapies, including treatments with antibiotics.
- stress - a major cause of many disorders in the intestine and is not only their own stress. The concept of the brain-gut axis is perfect to explain the role of stress in SIBO
- dysmotility - occurs when some of the muscles of the digestive system become lazy, or inactive. For this reason it is no longer able to remedy what has been digested, which remains in the small intestine. Once the intestine has good motility, it prevents microorganisms from sticking to the wall of the small intestine. If this does not happen, the bacteria

instead of going to the large intestine proliferate in the small intestine feeding on what has not been eliminated.

- intestinal inflammation - when the bowel is inflamed, it is for irritable bowel syndrome, Crohn's disease, the RCU or any other similar condition, the probability of suffering from SIBO is greater.
- birth control pills - it seems that the use of birth control pills is one of the causes of some intestinal inflammations, such as irritable bowel syndrome and Crohn's disease, and therefore, may be one of the causes of SIBO.
- antibiotics - Overuse of antibiotics leads on the one hand the development of pathogenic bacteria resistant to antibiotics and this is a serious health threat. On the other eliminates some 'good' bacteria that help us defend against pathogens, then prepares a perfect environment for the imbalance of which spoke initially which can lead to SIBO.
- alcohol consumption - some studies indicate SIBO among the causes of moderate alcohol consumption. The latter seems to have both on the intestinal motility, both on intestinal permeability. It also seems that food can specifically certain bacteria and this can lead to their excessive growth.

Functional Gastrointestinal Disorders (Fgid)

With this designation will include all those conditions in which the normal motor functions and digestive sensitivity are altered, but the origin of which are unable to highlight an organic cause. These functional alterations can afflict every digestive tract, esophagus, stomach, small intestine and colon.

These disorders are characterized by unpredictable symptoms and have strongly debilitating effects on the quality of life of sufferers.

From the scientific literature shows that 15-20% of the population in Western countries there is an affected, although FGID have spread to all continents. Women are more affected than men (2: 1) while all the age groups may suffer, including children from the age schoolchildren.

Although FGID are not associated in any way to deterioration of the body or to a shortening of life, they determine a considerable worsening of the same quality of life, with more and more frequent use of medical visits, diagnostic tests, drugs of any kind and sometimes also to unnecessary if not worsening surgeries. The FGID are the second leading cause of absenteeism from work after the flu.

No structural abnormality is present in the routine diagnostic tests; laboratory tests and radiological and endoscopic are normal. The diagnosis is as they say of "exclusion."

It is based on a careful assessment of the subjective and objective symptoms, after excluding organic diseases through the instrumental laboratory examinations.

The symptoms are:
- Heartburn or heartburn retrosternal resistant to all common antisecretory drugs (PPI).
- Chest pain retrosternal not due to heart problems.
- Dysphagia or difficult swallowing, both at the level of the throat of the chest.

- Dyspepsia or slow and difficult digestion (nausea, belching, headache post prandial, abdominal pain).
- Cyclic vomiting syndrome or recurrent and debilitating episodes of intense nausea and vomiting lasting for several hours, or days.
- Abdominal pain, continuous or recurring frequently.
- Irritable Bowel Syndrome: abdominal pain with marked swelling and disorders of intestinal emptying such as constipation and chronic diarrhea.

The various therapeutic attempts by family doctors or specialists will not go into these specific issues are almost always crowned with failure. In fact there is no standardized treatment for these disorders, but the medical specialist in this be packing industry a regimen of "personalized" which will include a qualitative diet (that is, excluding the foods that can trigger and / or maintain the symptoms), drugs that act at the level the lumen of the digestive tract, drugs that act at the level of the muscles of the digestive tract, drugs that act at the level of the enteric nervous system and peripheral for the last drugs that act at the level of the central nervous system.

Finally, practical life tips to combat constipation, diarrhea, nausea and vomiting, and to create empathy with the patient convince him that disturbances as unpleasant and debilitating not in any way compromise his health.

The Bloating, Abdominal Distension The Gas And Intestinal

Abdominal swelling: It can be defined as the unpleasant feeling that there is a bulging ball in our belly. It 'a symptom often reported by patients and is sometimes associated with distention, ie the visible increase in the area comprised between the hips and the cost, commonly called waistline. Swelling and distention causing discomfort and sometimes pain, impacting negatively on the quality of everyday life.

These two symptoms are associated with other disorders related to intestinal gas, such as belching, aerophagia (swallowing air), and the gas from the anus dumping (bloating and flatulence).

In people with functional gastrointestinal disorders bloating and distension are often up to 90% in the irritable bowel syndrome, in 50% in functional dyspepsia and in 56% of chronic constipation.

There is no certainty about the origin of these symptoms. The possible reasons are:

- Too much gas in the intestines.
- Excess of bacteria in the small intestine (Small Intestinal Bacterial Overgrowth-SIBO).
- Imbalance between the varieties of bacteria normally present in the intestine (dysbiosis), in particular after an antibiotic treatment.
- Food intolerance.
- Increased sensitivity and perception of what is happening in the gut.

- Increasing the curvature of the lumbar region of the spine (lumbar lordosis), which decreases the abdomen capacity to hold gas.
- Gastroparesis (complication of diabetes).

Each person has the gas in its digestive tract whether it is the esophagus, the stomach, the small intestine and the colon (or large intestine).

The gas can enter from outside the body, it can be produced inside of it, moves in the various areas of the digestive tract and is finally ejected.

The gas emission is a "normal" event, this does not squirmed can be an embarrassing fact or cause discomfort.

The gas enters in the following ways:

- Swallowing air. One part is ejected erupting, the remainder passes into the intestine.
- Passage of gas from the intestine blood.
- Production of gas from chemical reactions within the gut.
- food fermentation by intestinal bacteria.

  The gas is eliminated in the following ways:

- Erupting.
- Coming absorbed by the blood.
- Consumed by intestinal bacteria.
- Escaping from the anus (bloating and flatulence).
- Bacteria and intestinal gas.

The colon contains an enormous amount of bacteria. Some produce gas, while others consume.

Remnants of food that are not digested by enzymes in the small intestine content arrive in the colon where they are captured by the bacteria that produce gas; this process is called fermentation. In this way it is produced hydrogen (H) and carbon dioxide (CO_2). Other bacteria consume an enormous amount of hydrogen and release minor amounts of malodorous gases are methane and hydrogen sulphide. These are usually expelled from the anus.

And 'well it is known that the gas transits more quickly if a person is standing rather than lying down. If the gas stagnated inside the body there is a sense of tension and various other symptoms. They are better tolerated if the bowel is relaxed (ie is not spastic) and if the gas is in the colon rather than the small intestine.

Patients erupt very unintentionally swallow a lot of air that reaches the stomach and from there it is re-emitted. The solution is to prevent the intentional belching and decrease the maximum swallowing of air.

Heavy Breath (Halitosis), flatulence (gas too) and flatulence (smelly gas) are unsightly and sometimes embarrassing situations are due to the production of small amounts of hydrogen sulphide by specific colonic bacteria.

Some food substances increase the production of gas, these are:

- Fermentable fibers in the diet.
- Starches.
- Complex carbohydrates, which are the main cause, present in beans (some substances contained in the beans block the

enzymes that digest starches normally, so the starches pass without being digested in the colon where they are fermented by bacteria with an increase in gas production).

- Some sugars such as sorbitol and fructose.
- The cellulose contained in some plants.

Most people have no problem to remove excess gas, others suffer from this problem for psychological reasons or for bad coordination of the abdominal muscles.

The bad coordination of the abdominal muscles is also the basis of constipation which in turn increases the fermentation and thus the production of even smelling gas.

Belching and bloating

The air is ingested by eating or talking. Therefore speak or eat quickly or even worse, talk and eat simultaneously may underlie of aerophagia.

They also want to delete the chewing gum, smoking, and dentures shaky.

Bloating and flatulence

The power supply must be modified as they are the carbohydrate-based foods poorly digestible major responsible for these alterations of digestive functions, while fats and proteins are not responsible.

Foods that cause gas:
- Refined sugars, beans contain large amounts of this complex sugar; cabbage, brussel sprouts, broccoli, asparagus, other vegetables and whole grains contain albeit in smaller quantities.

- Lactose is the natural sugar in milk. It is also found in cheese, ice cream, bread, cereals and some seasoning sauces.
- Fructose, it is present in onions, artichokes, pears, wheat and corn. It is also added as a sweetener in many drinks and fruit juices.
- Sorbitol, it occurs naturally in fruits, such as apples, pears, peaches, and plums. It, too, is used as a sweetener in many foods low calorie or diet and sugar-free candy and chewing gum.
- Starch is present in potatoes, corn, noodles and wheat, and wheat. Coming digested by bacteria in the colon is the main gas agent. The rice has a starch that does not produce gas.
- Fibers, should be divided into soluble, ie which dissolve easily in water and insoluble. The soluble are digested only in the colon and its bacteria and thus produce gas. They are present in oat bran, beans, barley, nuts, seeds, lentils, peas, and many fruits. The insoluble fibers pass practically free throughout the bowel and therefore produce little gas. They are present in wheat bran, whole grains, and some vegetables.
- Alcohol, it can reduce the digestion in the gut, so that a greater amount of undigested food reaches the colon where it is fermented.
- Fats, it is better to restrict them as they slow down the gastro-intestinal emptying. If the stomach and intestines empty too vigorously, the gas is expelled more quickly.

To prevent and treat bloating the main nutritional claims about foods to avoid and some dietary advice - conduct to be followed during meals and throughout the day.

Dietary Recommendations:

- Eat meals at regular intervals
- Eat slowly and chew well
- Avoid talking while eating
- Avoid overeating
- No smoking especially during meals
- Avoid swallowing repeated (not chewing gum and candy)
- Before lying down after a meal, wait at least an hour has elapsed.
- Avoid drinking through a straw or a bottle with a narrow neck
- Practicing with physical activity regularly and always maintain an active lifestyle. It is always to be recommended to many and good reasons. In this case the tension and contraction of the abdominal muscles help to progression of the gas in the intestines, and then to its expulsion.
- Supplements, Tablets containing alpha-galactosidase by interfering at the beginning of the meal may be useful to prevent the formation of gas by bacterial fermentation.
- To the smell of copper salts and chlorophyll.
- At the pharmacy or herbal medicine, there are some herbal products that can be taken as teas or dietary supplements that help eliminate intestinal gas and bloating contrast:

anise, caraway, cranberry, mint, chamomile, myrtle, lemon balm, fennel, apple.

- Drugs, you should always consult with a good gastroenterologist before taking medications also counter (without a prescription). Drugs that stimulate bowel motility help to expel the gas.

Foods that cause gas:

- Beans (before putting them in soaking and cooking them with new water reduces the power of forming gas). fresh and dried legumes (beans, chickpeas, lentils, peas, lupines, soybean) in large quantities, also in soups or stews
- Avoid vegetables like artichokes, asparagus, broccoli, cabbage, Brussels sprouts, cauliflower, cucumber, green pepper, onions, radishes, parsley, cabbage carrots, cauliflower, Brussels sprouts, cabbage, turnip, onion, carrot, eggplant, radishes, cucumbers, peppers.
- Avoid fruits like plums, grapes, bananas, apples, chestnuts, peaches, raisins, bananas, apricots, plums, pears. unripe and dried fruit (walnuts, hazelnuts, pistachios, almonds)
- bran and whole grain, and gradually added with measure may reduce the formation of gas. Whole foods (bread, pasta, cookies, crackers, biscuits, bread sticks) in large quantities
- Bread-crumbs
- Spices and spicy foods (eg. Strong cheeses)
- Avoid carbonated drinks, especially sweet. Carbonated drinks (carbonated water, coke, sprite, orange juice, tonic water ...

- The carbonated mineral water is less annoying and for some it can however be helpful to digestion.
- Avoid milk, milk fresh cheese and spicy cheeses and ice cream
- latte, cappuccino, whipped cream, milk shakes and smoothies with or without milk ice cream, eggnog, creams and mousses
- packed Snacks prepared with lactose, milk bread, cereal, and salad dressings.
- Food or beverages that contain sorbitol like candy and chewing sugarless chewing King. Artificial sweeteners: sorbitol, xylitol, mannitol (also present in some candies and chewing-gum)
- Cocoa, milk chocolate, dark chocolate, hot chocolate
- Sauces: mayonnaise, cocktail sauce, mustard
- Avoid the following combinations of foods: meat and cheese; eggs and legumes; fresh pasta and bread.
- Avoid fatty and fried foods (fried vegetables, breaded and fried cheese, fried fish)
- Moderate wine and beer and avoid the black stuff.

Foods that produce bad breath and flatulence

- Alcohol, asparagus, beans, cabbage, chicken, coffee, cucumber, dairy, eggs, fish, garlic, nuts, onions, prunes, radishes, and highly seasoned foods.

Foods that produce little gas

- Meat, poultry, fish.

- Eggs.
- Vegetables such as lettuce, tomatoes, zucchini.
- Fruits such as melon, grapes, strawberries, raspberries, blueberries, blackberries, currants and all berries, cherries, avocados, olives.
- Carbohydrates gluten, rice bread and rice.

Also recommended is the diet LOW-FODMAP and its two-phase system, the first and the second elimination of reintegration.

The response to changes in supply varies from person to person. Try deleting a week foods and drinks that seem suspicious to produce gas or odor. Then reintroduce them one at a time to identify which of them produces the symptoms.

All have intestinal gas. It can be annoying and cause embarrassment in social life, but it is not a situation of disease.

To control it the best you have to pay attention to dentures too much furniture that result in an increase of air swallowed with the saliva.

Problems of chronic inflammation of the nose and paranasal sinuses lead to increased swallowing so much air that enters the stomach.

Smoking cigars or pipe increases saliva ingested and with it the air.

Avoid eating quickly, talking eating, chewing gum and sucking on candy or lollipops.

Crohn's Disease

Crohn's disease is chronic intestinal inflammation that can affect the entire gastrointestinal tract. The causes are still unknown. It is characterized by intestinal ulcers, often alternating with stretches of healthy intestine, and, if not treated properly, can lead to complications such as stenosis or fistulas that may require surgery. Symptoms can range from abdominal pain, chronic diarrhea, to weight loss or fever.

In about 90% of cases, the disease mostly affects the last part of the small intestine (ileum) and the colon.

Ulcers derived inflammation, if left untreated, can lead to create intestinal narrowing (stenosis) or deepening up to "pierce" the gut and touch the surrounding organs (fistulas). These complications often require surgical treatment, although the disease can come back at the point where surgical resection is performed. Nevertheless, the majority of patients, with care and necessary controls, can well control the disease and lead a regular life.

The causes

The causes of the disease are unknown. It seems that a combination of factors, such as genetic predisposition, environmental factors, cigarette smoking, and alterations of intestinal flora and the immune response, can trigger intestinal inflammation. In fact, the cells of the immune system "attacks" continuously the intestine and help perpetuate inflammation. Although some genes appear to be involved, it is not a hereditary disease, or genetic.

The symptoms of Crohn's disease

Crohn's disease can manifest itself in different ways depending on the intestinal localizations. The most common symptoms are chronic diarrhea (ie which persists for more than 4 weeks), often at night, associated with abdominal pain and cramps, sometimes with mixed blood loss to the stool, and low-grade fever that occurs in the evening, or with joint pain, or other non-intestinal manifestations. Often there can be a significant drop in weight. Sometimes, you can manifest in level with anal fistulas or collections of pus (abscess).

In a large percentage of cases, the disease has no symptoms and is discovered only by accident.

Diagnosis

The methods for diagnosing Crohn's disease are:

- The colonoscopy with ileum and visualization with intestinal biopsy: is used to assess the state of the intestinal mucosa and to assess whether, at the microscopic level, there are typical aspects of chronic inflammation (structural alterations of the tissue, infiltrated white blood cells). It is essential for diagnosis.
- Ultrasonography of the intestinal loops: allows to evaluate the intestinal wall noninvasively, to rule out or diagnose complications from the disease.
- The abdominal magnetic resonance imaging with contrast medium that allows you to locate the inflammation, to assess any complications and to evaluate the extent and inflammatory activity. It is a noninvasive procedure that does not expose to harmful rays.

- The endoscopic enteroscopy is a non-invasive method to diagnose injuries of the small intestine that are not accessible by colonoscopy. It is limited by the impossibility of doing biopsies and the risk of retention, in case of intestinal stenosis.
- Surgical exploration under anesthesia is a surgical technique that is used in selected cases of perianal Crohn's disease. It is with diagnostic and curative.

Treatments

Treatment for Crohn's disease tends to shut down the intestinal inflammation through action on the cellular and molecular mechanisms of the intestine and immune system. It must be prescribed by the doctor based on the patient's symptoms.

Prevention

Unfortunately we can't prevent the onset of Crohn's disease, but it can prevent complications and evolution.

- Early detection of disease is to require blood tests, stool and a non-invasive examination of the abdomen (ultrasound or CT or MRI) in case of diarrhea and / or abdominal pain persists for more than four weeks, weight loss, symptoms nightlife, especially in people with a family history of autoimmune diseases.
- Prevention of complications, performing blood tests and stool every 6-12 months, and a non-invasive examination of the abdomen (CT or MRI), ultrasound, at least annually, supplemented if necessary by a colonoscopy

- Prevention of intestinal neoplasia by performing a colonoscopy with serial biopsies every 12 months in the case of extended Crohn's disease in the colon, starting from 10 years of diagnosis
- Prevention of opportunistic infections in patients who are undergoing chronic immunosuppressive therapy for Crohn's disease, performing influenza vaccination every 12 months, anti-pneumococcal vaccination every 5 years, and vaccination for hepatitis B at the time of diagnosis if It not already carried out. In women, it is recommended in these cases, the HPV vaccination.

The Ulcerative Colitis

Ulcerative colitis, along with Crohn's disease, is part of the inflammatory bowel disease and consists of an inflammation of the intestinal wall, which persists over time (chronic) and causes diarrhea, often with blood, pain, weakness and weight loss . Inflammation develops starting from the last intestinal tract, the rectum, with the presence of superficial ulcers, and may extend the time until the initial portion of the colon that is located in the right part of the abdomen.

In relation to the extension of inflammation of the colon, ulcerative colitis is classified as:

- proctitis, if it affects only the rectum;
- if left colitis affects the rectum and descending colon (part of the intestine which is located in the left side of the abdomen);

- colitis extended, if the inflammation extends to the horizontal portion of the colon (the one that is located immediately below the stomach) and the ascending part which is located on the right side of the abdomen.

Inflammatory manifestations may occur in other parts of the body such as joints, skin and eye.

The disease is characterized by phases in which there are disturbances (symptoms) interspersed with periods in which they are completely absent or are mild (remission). Complications that can occur over time include very heavy bleeding and acute dilation of the colon.

The chronic inflammation also can help, over time, an increased risk of colorectal cancer. The current treatment strategies aim to avoid as far as possible, the appearance of such complications.

It can occur at any age, usually it appears in young adults even if a few years more and more cases occurring in children and adolescents. When the disease affects children can affect the growth process, both in the period prior to its discovery, both in the first year following his assessment (diagnosis).

Ulcerative colitis is not to be confused with the more common irritable bowel syndrome that causes disorders such as constipation, diarrhea, abdominal pain not associated with the presence of inflammation.

Symptoms

The intensity and type of disturbances caused by ulcerative colitis are related to the severity of inflammation and the affected part of the colon and may include:

- rid of urgency from feces (evacuation)
- feeling of incomplete evacuation (rectal tenesmus)
- bleeding from the rectum
- chronic diarrhea, often at night
- presence of blood and mucus in the stool
- constipation paradoxical, present in approximately 10% of patients with involvement of the rectum and descending colon (proctitis and left colitis)
- abdominal pains
- weight loss
- fatigue
- temperature
- loss of appetite
- in children, growth slowdown

The presence of bloody diarrhea, pain and weight loss are the association of disorders (symptoms) can appear more frequently, but even some of them. The inflammation of the rectum (ulcerative proctitis) is often characterized by urgent evacuation, tenesmus and bleeding, and fever, feeling tired and weight loss are associated more frequently with extensive colitis. In some cases it can occur even vomiting. The disorders (symptoms) may occur intermittently with periods in which they are present (exacerbations) alternating with periods of total absence (remission).

You should consult your doctor if you experience a persistent and repeated changes over time in bowel habits or if you have aliments such as:

- abdominal pain
- blood in the stool
- lasting diarrhea (at least 4 weeks)
- diarrhea night
- Repeated fever (recurrent) with no apparent cause

Causes

The cause of ulcerative colitis are not yet clear. The currently available knowledge lead you to think that developments due to improper stimulation of the body's defense system (immune system) determined by environmental factors (including diet) that act on the intestinal microbial flora of people genetically predisposed. It was also hypothesized the presence of some agents that can cause disease but there is no definitive evidence.

The factors involved in the development of the disease are:

- genetic factors, there is a familial predisposition to develop the disease
- immunological factors, malfunction of the body's defense system (immune system) that reacts inappropriately towards the microorganisms normally present in the intestine (intestinal flora). Such action is favored by a defect of the intestinal mucosa which causes a greater entry of organisms

that make up the bacterial flora in the intestinal wall thickness
- environmental factors, the type diet "Western" would seem to favor the occurrence of disease. Environmental factors, in fact, would affect the composition of the bacterial flora resulting in a reduction in the number of microorganisms that protect the gut to the benefit of those who damage

Risk factors:

Ulcerative colitis is a disease that affects an equal number of both men and women. Risk factors may include:
- age, the disease affects, usually before the age of thirty, but in some cases, can occur even after 60 years
- race or ethnicity, whites have a higher risk of getting sick but ulcerative colitis can occur in any breed. The Ashkenazi Jews have a higher risk
- families already affected by the disease (family history), the risk of illness is greater if you have a first-degree relative already ill

Diagnosis

The assessment of early stage disease (early diagnosis) allows you to immediately start caring more appropriate and to prevent the development of complications that may be irreversible.

There is no single test to identify ulcerative colitis, its finding is based on a combination of clinical, endoscopic examinations, histological and radiological analysis, complemented by a careful assessment of the person's state of health history that suffers.

The diagnosis also serves to rule out other diseases that may present with the same disorders such as, for example, Crohn's disease, or SIBO.

For the investigation (diagnosis) of ulcerative colitis are performed a series of tests which include:

- Blood tests, such as blood count
- stool tests (bacterial culture and parasitological stool)
- colonoscopy, indispensable examination to detect (diagnose) ulcerative colitis, allows not only to highlight the intestinal lesions but also to take small fragments of tissue (biopsies) on which to carry out the histological examination
- abdomen radiography, at the present time is executed if it is suspected the presence of toxic megacolon premegacolon and to evaluate the distribution of the intestinal gas. With the progress of endoscopic techniques, however, the examination has lost much of the importance of diagnostic who had prior to endoscopy
- abdominal ultrasound, to assess the state of the intestinal wall noninvasively
- Computerized axial tomography (CT) of the abdomen

The imaging studies, particularly abdominal ultrasound, should be performed in hospitals with experience in the assessment (diagnosis) and treatment of chronic inflammatory bowel disease.

Lifestyle

Often you may feel powerless in the face of ulcerative colitis. But changes in diet and lifestyle can help control the symptoms and lengthen the time between exacerbations. There is no direct scientific evidence that what you eat actually causes an inflammatory bowel disease. But some foods and drinks can worsen the signs and symptoms, especially during disease flare. It may be helpful to keep a food diary to keep track of what you are eating, and how it feels. If you find that certain foods are causing particular symptoms, you can try to eliminate them. Here are some tips that may help:

- Limit dairy products. Many people with inflammatory bowel disease note that problems such as diarrhea, abdominal pain and swelling improve by limiting or eliminating dairy products. It may also be lactose intolerant (your body can not digest the milk sugar, lactose), but this is a chronic condition, in the case of inflammatory bowel disease such symptoms can occur only in the exacerbation phases.
- Try foods low in fat. In the case of Crohn's disease of the small intestine, you might not be able to digest or absorb fat normally. So, fats pass through the intestine, making diarrhea worse. Avoid butter, margarine, and cream and fried foods.
- Limit the use of fiber. In the case of inflammatory bowel disease, high fiber foods, such as fresh fruits and vegetables and whole grains, can make symptoms worse. If raw fruits and vegetables cause discomfort, try steaming or stewing. In general, you may have more problems with the cabbage family foods, such as broccoli and cauliflower, and nuts, seeds, corn and popcorn. Using a low-residue diet fiber if there is a narrowing of the intestine (sub-stenosis).

- Avoid spicy foods. Alcohol and caffeine can worsen the signs and symptoms of the disease.
- Eat small meals. Patients report being better in making five or six small meals a day instead of two or three more abundant.
- Drink plenty of fluids. Try to drink plenty of fluids a day. Water is best. Alcohol and beverages that contain caffeine to stimulate bowel motility and can make diarrhea worse, while carbonated drinks frequently produce gas.
- Consider using multivitamins. Because inflammatory bowel disease may interfere with the ability to absorb some nutrients and given that diet may be limited, the 'use of multivitamins and minerals is often useful. Consult with your doctor before taking any vitamin or supplement.
- Talk to a dietitian. If you start to lose weight or diet has become very limited, according to the gastroenterologist should consult dietitian
- A proven risk factor linked to lifestyle is smoking, so if you smoke you need to quit smoking.

Celiac Disease

Celiac disease is a genetic disease and inflammatory nature characterized principally by the destruction of the mucosa (surface part) of the small intestine.

It is caused by an immune reaction to gluten, a term used generically to indicate some specific proteins of wheat, barley and rye. Foods that contain these grains are numerous and are extremely popular on the tables of Italian bread, pizza, pasta and biscuits.

The symptoms with which it presents the celiac disease can be very different, to be borne by different organs and different severity. Furthermore, celiac disease may begin at any age, even in old age.

Celiac disease is associated, often in the same individual to other autoimmune diseases, such as type 1 diabetes, rheumatoid arthritis, thyroid disease, but also to genetic syndromes (Down's syndrome and Turner's syndrome).

The causes

In people genetically predisposed to celiac disease, the cells of the immune system, triggered by contact with gluten, attack the mucosa of the small intestine. In this way they destroy the villi (the villi are small finger-shaped protrusions, responsible for the absorption of various nutrients and minerals that, through the wall of the small intestine, end up in the blood). They determine malabsorption and malnutrition.

The causes for the development of celiac disease are:
- the environmental factor, follow a cereal-based diet containing gluten;
- the genetic factor, being genetically predisposed. This means the presence of specific sequences in the genes, which define the structure with which our immune cells, in this way they in fact recognize the different elements that come into contact with them.

The National Institute of Diabetes and Digestive and Kidney Diseases, claims that breastfeeding seems to play a protective role, a self-defense, or at least seems to delay its onset.

Currently it is estimated that celiac disease affects around 1% of the general population and is more common among women (three times more than men).

In fact, although it is one of the most frequent chronic diseases, in reality there are still several hundred thousand people with celiac disease to diagnose.

Symptoms

The symptoms of celiac disease are extremely variable per location and intensity.

In the so-called celiac disease CLASSICAL FORM (usually with DEBUT FROM CHILDREN) dominate the symptoms and signs of malabsorption:

- incidents of foul-smelling diarrhea (due to the presence of fat in the stool)
- meteorism (swollen abdomen) also marked,
- crampy abdominal pain
- poor growth.

The classic form of celiac disease has become increasingly rare and frequently celiac disease manifests itself in ADULT with extra-intestinal nonspecific symptoms (also known as ATYPICAL SYMPTOMS). Often, however, these symptoms are mild and the correct diagnosis requires years. Among these:

- iron deficiency anemia,

- osteoporosis,
- muscle weakness;
- disorders of fertility and repeated miscarriages,
- coagulation disorders,
- oral aphthae,
- alopecia,
- tingling on the hands and feet,
- convulsions.

The disease can also manifest with symptoms of the diseases associated with it: autoimmune thyroid disease, type 1 diabetes, psoriasis, gastritis, autoimmune hepatitis, and, above all, herpetiformis Duhring dermatitis, characterized by vesicles extremely itchy appearing on the surface of the legs, back and buttocks.

The diagnosis

For a diagnosis of celiac disease, well-defined guidelines must be followed.

There are subjects who may be more predisposed than others. In cases of celiac disease due to familiarity, the appearance of symptoms referable to it or the presence of a frequently associated disease, the first test performed (using a simple blood test) is the dosage of specific antibodies produced in the blood in response to the presence of gluten. As in most blood tests, the patient on an empty stomach. To detect the presence of anti-TG Ig antibodies in the blood, a pharmacy test is also available, with a kit similar to that used for diabetes monitoring, at a cost that varies between 30 and $ 60. If the result is positive , we proceed to investigate the presence of celiac disease.

Patients who have all or some of these antibodies are subjected to biopsy (a sample of a tissue fragment is taken) of the first part of the small intestinal mucosa, the duodenum, in order to document a flattening (disappearance) of the intestinal villi.

Genetic analysis, carried out through DNA testing, reveals whether you are predisposed to the disease. However, this test must be reserved only for those subjects, in which the antibody test, the duodenal biopsy and the symptoms are not completely clear.

Given its characteristic genetic transmission, it is advisable in the family to screen antibodies to the patient's first-degree relatives.

Therapy

Unfortunately, to date the only therapy currently available for celiac disease is the exclusion from the diet of all possible sources of gluten (often lastingly), including those that can contain it (gluten can be present in canned foods, in packaged soups, in sauces, but also in cosmetics and medicines. It can be used as an additive, preservative or flavoring).

Normally, the gluten-free diet (gluten-free) causes rapid disappearance of symptoms and remission of the disappearance of the villi of the duodenal mucosa.

The resilience and recovery of damaged tissues, however, also depends on many other factors such as, for example, the age at which the disease is diagnosed, the amount of damage or the assumption by individuals of other drugs which can interfere.

If the diet is respected and the disease is in its early stages, a significant improvement of the clinical picture usually occurs within a few weeks of starting a gluten-free diet, while the total resolution of symptoms may take several months. The time required for complete reconstitution of the intestinal mucosa depend on the degree of damage and the age of the patient: in adults, in fact, it can take up to 2 years of gluten-free diet for the full restoration of the intestinal villi.

Following a gluten-free diet is necessary to prevent complications of celiac disease; in fact, if it is not promptly diagnosed and treated in an appropriate manner, this may lead to the development of other diseases, such as:

- lymphomas and adenocarcinomas,
- forms of bowel cancer,
- osteoporosis (arising from poor absorption of calcium),
- miscarriages and birth defects (during pregnancy, the intake of nutrients is particularly crucial for good health of the fetus)
- short stature (especially when the celiac disease develops in childhood and does not allow, therefore, an adequate absorption of nutrients necessary for growth),
- convulsions and seizures (derived from deposition of calcium in the brain as a result of a deficiency of folic acid to poor absorption).

The gluten-free diet

Choosing to start following a gluten-free diet means having to eliminate from your diet, potentially all foods derived from wheat, barley and other cereals, and therefore almost all packaged foods: from snacks to cakes, from pasta, with bread and pizza. The meat, vegetables, rice, corn and potatoes however, they do not contain gluten and, therefore, may be part of the celiac diet.

WARNING! GLUTEN-FREE DIET MUST BE FOLLOWED ONLY IN CASE OF DIAGNOSED CELIAC!

Those who choose to eat gluten free, while not suffering from celiac disease, is exposed to the risk of getting diabetes.

Gluten-free diets have become very popular in recent years. Surely this choice of food is good for those who suffer from intolerance to the molecule, or to celiacs. But let's not forget, the Harvard University study in Boston shows that this diet increases the risk of diabetes by 13%. These results were presented at the American Heart Association meeting, conducted on 200,000 people followed for 30 years.

Chapter 4: the low-fodmap diet cookbook for breakfast

Cocoa Pancake

For two people:
- 1 ripe banana (100 gr)
- 60 grams of rice flour
- 2 teaspoons of cocoa
- 2 eggs
- 50 ml of almond or rice milk
- a little bit of baking soda

To garnish:
- Peanut butter

Direction:

- To mix all the ingredients use a food processor until they are well combined.
- Let the dough rest for 10/15 minutes.
- Put some butter or oil in a pan. Warm it up.
- Slowly pour a spoonful of batter into small pancakes.
- Cook the pancake for about 35 seconds on both sides.
- Serve the pancakes by adding peanut butter.

Banana Bread

Ingredients for a 20 cm bread

- 130 grams of flour (buckwheat)
- 3 ripe bananas
- 50 grams of extra-virgin olive oil
- 8 gr of baking powder
- A little bit of salt
- Vanilla powder

Instructions

- Heat the oven to a temperature of 170 ° C.
- Blend the bananas until they form a cream.
- Add the eggs to the bananas, add the extra-virgin olive oil and stir until a soft dough is created. Better if you use an electric mixer.
- , Mix the flour in a medium-sized bowl. Baking powder, salt and vanilla powder.
- Add the dry ingredients (flour, yeast, salt and vanilla powder) to the others (eggs, bananas and oil).
- At this point it is important to mix well with a wooden spoon. Follow the direction from bottom to top.
- Put the mixture in a 20 cm* pan with parchment paper.
- Cook in a ventilated oven for about 45 minutes or until completely cooked, checking the cooking with a wooden stick.
- Season with yogurt and fruit.
- You can keep the bread in a closed container for 2/3 days.

Notes

* The baking tray must be of the indicated size, otherwise you risk not to cook the dough well.

Carrot Cake Coconut Porridge

Ingredients

- 40 grams of rice flakes
- 180 ml of almond milk without sugar
- 15 gr of coconut butter
- 30 grams of finely grated carrots
- 1 teaspoon of maple syrup
- Vanilla powder

Instructions to be followed in two phases:

- Put the rice flakes in a bowl with 100 ml of almond milk the night before. Put in the fridge with a lid and let it rest during the night. Thanks to this the rice flakes will become softer.
- The following morning, add to the flakes of rice, coconut butter, maple syrup, carrots, vanilla powder and the remaining almond milk.
- Mix well and cook over very low heat. Continue cooking for a few minutes until the porridge is thick and creamy.

Notes

* To prepare coconut butter at home. Put a little dried grated coconut in a blender until creamy (about 12 minutes). Make it remarry and once it has cooled down, it will become solid. If too solid you can make it creamy again by heating it. Therefore, we

can replace coconut butter with a normal chopped dried coconut, but in this case the porridge will be less creamy.

Carrot Cake Cookies

It produces around 14 biscuits

- 100 grams of oat porridge (gluten free, if necessary)
- 85 grams of gluten-free flour mixture *
- 75 grams of grated carrots (1 medium-large carrot)
- 80 ml of maple syrup
- 3 tablespoons of extra-virgin olive oil
- 1 egg
- 2 teaspoons of raisins (only if appreciated) **
- 1 and a half teaspoon of baking powder
- A little bit of salt
- Vanilla powder

Instructions

- Allow the oven to warm up (preferably ventilated) to a temperature of 170/180 ° C.
- In a medium-large bowl, combine and mix the gluten-free flour mixture, porridge oats, baking powder, salt and vanilla powder.
- In another medium-large bowl, beat the egg maple syrup icon and oil using a whisk.
- To this second mixture, add the grated carrots and finally the other dry ingredients. Mix well for a few minutes.

- Put the mixture in the refrigerator for about 12/15 minutes. In this way, the mixture will become denser.
- Next, divide the dough into 14 scoops and form flat balls. You can flatten them using a fork or the back of a spoon.
- Put the cookies in the oven for about 20 minutes or until they turn golden.
- You can store them in an airtight container for about 3 days.

Notes

* You can use 55 grams of rice flour and 30 grams of potato starch.

** Up to 1 tablespoon of raisins is LOW-FODMAP, but not eating more than 5 biscuits.

Our cookies are different

When you start looking for them, you will realize that it is not easy to find LOW-FODMAP cookies on the market. It is not enough in fact that they are gluten-free, it is also necessary to check that they do not contain lactose, honey or agave, lupine flour, glucose-fructose syrup. If, in addition to LOW-FODMAPs, you also look for the quality of the ingredients and then try to avoid additives and preservatives, society becomes even more difficult.

But even prepared gluten-free desserts are not easy: unfortunately, no gluten-free flour perfectly replaces that of wheat, so it is often necessary to ensure small tricks to avoid getting desserts that are not compact or slightly leavened.

For example, the use of maple syrup in recipes offers many advantages. From a nutritional point of view there are no big differences between one and the other, they are always sugars, so it is necessary to consume them in moderation (including maple syrup).

The reasons for using maple syrup are: in addition to having a delicious taste, it makes the dough much more compact and less grainy. In this case, even honey could be an excellent substitute for sin which is high FODMAP.

But if you don't want to buy maple syrup because it costs too much, you can replace it with rice, which tastes less good, but has a very similar consistency.

The biscuits we have proposed are a review of the classic carrot biscuits, very popular in England and the United States. These biscuits have a soft and slightly spongy texture, so they look like small cakes.

In this recipe the biscuits are enriched with a bit of raisins, which in this diet should be consumed in moderation (maximum 1 tablespoon per meal). Even in this case, do not overdo it. If you prefer, you can still replace it with chocolate chips or simply omit it.

Green Smoothie Bowl With Chia Pudding

Ingredients for 1 bowl

For the chia pudding

- 130 ml of almond milk (without sugar)
- 15 grams of chia seeds
- 1 teaspoon of maple syrup
- Vanilla powder

For the smoothie

- 130 ml of almond milk without sugar
- 1 banana, small and ripe
- A handful of spinach
- 1 teaspoon of walnut butter (type to taste)

Two-step procedure:

- The evening before (or 6 hours before) peel the banana and after having cut it into slices, place it in an airtight container and then in the freezer.
- In a jar, mix chia seeds with 130 ml of almond milk, maple syrup and vanilla. Put the jar in the refrigerator.
- The next morning, put the remaining 130 ml of almond milk, the still-frozen banana, spinach and nut butter in a blender. Blend until it forms a cream
- If the dough is too thick and it is difficult to mix it, you can add some almond milk.
- In a medium-large bowl, first pour the smoothie and add the chia pudding.

Desert Petals

Ingredients for 16 biscuits

- 80 grams of rice flour
- 28 grams of potato starch
- 50 grams of white almonds
- 1 teaspoon (about 4 grams) of baking powder
- 1 egg

- 70 grams of raw cane sugar
- 75 grams of clarified butter
- Gluten-free corn flakes

Instructions

- Heat the oven (preferably ventilated) at a temperature of 170/180 °C.
- Grind the almonds with a food processor.
- In a medium-large bowl, mix the rice flour with the potato starch, chopped almonds and baking powder.
- Beat the butter with the egg and sugar. Use an electric whisk.
- Insert the dry ingredients at this point and mix well for a few minutes.
- Shape the balls and cover them completely with the corn flakes.
- Put the parchment paper on a baking sheet and then add it.. Cook for about 18 minutes.

Notes

Simple and tasty biscuits. The dough is very simple, based on flour, eggs, butter and sugar. The biscuits are enriched with chopped almonds, which make them soft. Corn flakes add a bit of "crunchiness".

Buckwheat And Coconut Granola

Ingredients

- 120 grams of buckwheat flakes
- 40/50 grams of grated and dried coconut
- 60 grams of mixed nuts and seeds (almonds, hazelnuts, walnuts or pumpkin seeds)
- 2 tablespoons of extra virgin coconut oil (30 gr)
- 1 tablespoon of maple syrup
- A little vanilla powder

Instructions

- Place the buckwheat flakes on a tray (place the parchment paper on the tray first).
- Put the grated coconut and mix well.
- Chop (not too much) nuts and add them to buckwheat and coconut flakes.
- Add the vanilla powder.
- In a medium-sized saucepan, melt the coconut oil and then add the maple syrup.
- Combine all the ingredients and mix well for a few minutes, until everything is well combined.
- Bake at 160 ° C for about 17 minutes or until the mixture turns golden.

Note

In this recipe there is the combination of coconut and buckwheat. A muesli prepared with buckwheat and grated coconut flakes.

Buckwheat (without peel) has been tested and is LOW-FODMAP, as is flour. Unfortunately, the buckwheat flakes have not yet been tested, but they will probably also be considered LOW-FODMAP.

Crispy Chocolate Quinoa Bars

Ingredients for 7 bars

- 120 grams of mixed nuts
- 9 tablespoons of quinoa flakes
- 2 tablespoons of maple syrup
- 30 grams of dark chocolate
- Vanilla powder

Instructions

- Chop the dark chocolate into many pieces.
- Using the food processor, mix the nuts until you get a sticky mixture.
- In a medium-large bowl, combine the walnut paste obtained, maple syrup, quinoa flakes, vanilla powder. Mix well for a few minutes
- Add dark chocolate.
- Spread the dough on a baking sheet (place the parchment paper on top), forming a rectangle.

- Cut the dough to form 7 strips. Use a sharp knife.
- Heat the oven to 160 ° C. Cook for about 30 minutes or until the bars are golden brown.

Notes

To prepare coconut bars, you can replace two tablespoons of quinoa flakes with 2 tablespoons of grated coconut (so it will be 6 tablespoons of quinoa flakes + 2 tablespoons of grated coconut).

You can also replace quinoa flakes with other types of cereal flakes, such as oats or buckwheat flakes.

Pumpkin Pancakes

Ingredients for mini-pancakes 8/10

- 60 grams of oatmeal
- 2 eggs
- 120 grams of pumpkin, steamed and pureed
- 50 ml of almond milk (without sugar)
- 1 tablespoon of maple syrup
- a pinch of baking powder
- Vanilla powder
- A pinch of extra-virgin coconut oil (or clarified butter)

Instructions

- In a medium-large bowl, mix the oatmeal, baking powder and vanilla powder.

- In a large bowl, beat the eggs with the maple syrup and the pumpkin puree, slowly add the almond milk and continue to beat.
- Add the dry ingredients one at a time (oatmeal, baking powder and vanilla). Continue to stir.
- In a pan, melt some extra-virgin coconut oil (or ghee *).
- Pour a ladle of batter into the pan (hot) forming a small pancake. Cook for about 2 minutes.
- Turn it over and cook it on the other side for another minute.
- Perform the same procedure until the batter runs out.

Notes

* If you have good quality non-stick pans, you don't need to add butter or oil.

** Using pumpkin to make pancakes is an alternative that offers several advantages. Pumpkin is an important ingredient to make pancakes of the right consistency: that is soft, but at the same time compact. The pinch of baking powder contributes to making the pancakes even softer. If you think yeast can make you sick, you can omit it.

Pumpkin And Chocolate Chip Muffins

Ingredients for 9 muffins
- 60 gr rice flour *
- 60 gr of tapioca (or cornstarch or potatoes) *
- 60 grams of buckwheat flour *
- 85 grams of coconut sugar (or raw cane sugar) **

- 100 grams pumpkin, steamed
- 100 grams of coconut yoghurt (or lactose-free yogurt)
- 50 grams of extra-virgin coconut oil
- 3 teaspoons of baking powder
- 1 egg
- 60 grams of dark chocolate
- Vanilla powder

Instructions

- Chop dark chocolate into medium-sized pieces. You can also do it with a knife.
- In a medium-sized bowl, mix the flours (rice flour, tapioca and buckwheat flour), yeast, sugar, vanilla and chopped chocolate.
- Take a large bowl. Mix the egg with the pumpkin puree, yogurt and extra-virgin coconut. Use an electric mixer for a better result.
- Mix all the ingredients together.
- Transfer everything into muffin boxes. Cook at 170/180 ° C for about 35 minutes.

Notes

* You can also replace these flours with those without gluten.

** There are no certain data if coconut sugar is included among the FODMAPS. If you think you can't tolerate it, you can replace it with raw cane sugar.

Baked Millet Pudding With Pine Nuts

Ingredients for 2 small puddings

- 60 grams of millet
- 15 grams of almond butter (or hazelnuts)
- 1 tablespoon of maple syrup (or rice)
- 1 egg
- 1 tablespoon of pine nuts (or raisins)
- A banana (about 75 grams), crushed
- 75 ml of almond milk (without sugar)
- Vanilla powder
- Ghee or coconut oil

Instructions

- Cook the millet. You can cook it following the instructions on the package.
- Using a whisk, mix the almond butter, maple syrup and egg.
- Add some vanilla powder, the crushed banana and almond milk.
- Continue to stir for about a minute and a half.
- Add the cooked millet to this point.
- Insert the mixture into two greased cups. Put the pine nuts on top.
- Cook for 35 minutes at 160 ° C.

Notes

If you prefer, you can replace millet with rice.

Oat Porridge With Blueberry Coulis

Ingredients (1 portion)

- 40 grams of oats (choose organic and gluten-free) *
- 200 ml of almond milk without sugar (or 100 ml coconut milk and 100 ml coconut water)
- 1/2 banana, crushed
- Vanilla powder
- Blueberry coulis
- 300 grams of blueberries
- 1 tablespoon of Demerara sugar
- A little lemon juice
- 1/2 cup of water
- Vanilla powder
- Almond Butter
- Banana slices (optional)

Instructions

- Prepare the blueberry coulis. Put in a saucepan: blueberries, water, sugar, lemon juice and vanilla powder.
- Cook everything on low heat. Cook until the coulis has thickened (about 30 minutes).
- Prepare the porridge. Simmer oats and almond milk in a saucepan.

- Add the 1/2 crushed banana and vanilla powder.
- Continue stirring until it thickens (about 3 minutes).
- Serve seasoned with blueberry coulis and banana slices. If you prefer also almond cream.

Notes

* If you prefer buckwheat flakes or rice flakes, they require a longer cooking time. You should put them in water and half of the almond milk overnight to soften them. The next morning, heat them in a saucepan with the remaining almond milk, half a banana and vanilla powder.

Buckwheat - Coconut Biscuits

Ingredients for 12 biscuits

- 60 grams of rice flour
- 60 grams of buckwheat flour
- 25 grams of coconut flour (NOT grated coconut) *
- 75 grams of coconut oil
- 1/4 teaspoon baking powder
- 100 ml of coconut milk (or if you prefer almond milk)
- A pinch of vanilla powder

Instructions

- Dissolve the coconut oil by heating it
- In a medium-sized bowl, mix the rice flour, buckwheat flour and coconut flour. Combine and continue to mix the yeast and vanilla powder.

- Prepare melted coconut oil together with maple syrup in a bowl. Mix them for a few minutes.
- Combine the two mixtures and mix well using both hands.
- Slowly add the coconut milk. Mix well.
- Make balls of dough and flatten with a fork.
- Put them on a baking sheet (always place the parchment paper on top) and bake at 180 ° for about 23 minutes or until golden brown.

Notes

* Remember that coconut contains small amounts of FODMAP: and exactly polyol sorbitol. 4-5 cookies shouldn't give you problems. It is however better to consume these cookies not during the period of elimination of the diet, but during the subsequent reintroduction phase.

Be careful not to confuse coconut flour with grated coconut. Coconut flour is in fact produced from the dried coconut pulp.

Vanilla Millet Porridge

Ingredients for 1 portion

- 50 grams of millet
- 120 ml of coconut water (also good or just water) *
- 100 ml of whole coconut milk
- 2 teaspoons of maple syrup
- Vanilla powder

Indications

- First put the millet in a colander and rinse thoroughly.

- In a medium-sized saucepan, pour the water (coconut), and the millet. Cook over medium-low heat until all the water runs out.
- Add coconut milk, vanilla and maple syrup. Continue cooking for 7 minutes, stirring occasionally.
- If you have decided to prepare the millet the night before, put it in the refrigerator. The following morning, just heat the coconut milk in a saucepan, add the millet, maple syrup, vanilla and mix for a few minutes.
- Season porridge with fresh or dried fruit.

Notes

* Use coconut water to have more sweetness.

The FODMAP content of the millet has not yet been tested and is uncertain. It is certainly a very digestible cereal, it is gluten-free and rich in mineral salts. You can replace millet with other gluten-free grains like rice or buckwheat.

Chocolatey Overnight Chia And Banana Oats

Ingredients for a portion

- 30 grams of oat flakes (preferably small)
- 1 tablespoon of chia seeds
- 1 medium-sized banana
- 170 ml of unsweetened almond milk
- 1 teaspoon of maple syrup (if desired)
- 2 teaspoons of cocoa

- Vanilla powder

Toppings

- Almond Butter
- Grated coconut

Instructions

- Combine and blend the banana, almond milk, cocoa, maple syrup and vanilla powder.
- In a medium sized bowl mix oats and chia seeds.
- Add the banana and cocoa smoothie. Mix everything for a few minutes.
- Let the bowl rest in the fridge for one night (7 hours).
- In the morning you can make your breakfast more tasty by adding only almond butter or grated coconut.

Chestnut Pancakes With Raw Cocoa Spread

Ingredients for 2 people (about 10 mini-pancakes)

- 75 grams of chestnut flour
- 170 ml of almond milk without sugar
- 2 eggs
- 1 tablespoon of maple syrup
- Vanilla powder

For the spread of cocoa

- 1 banana
- 3 teaspoons of cocoa
- 1 tablespoon of almond butter (choose 100% almonds)

Instructions

- First, prepare the cream. Add banana, cocoa and almond butter in a blender. Work it until it becomes smooth.
- In a medium-sized bowl mix the chestnut flour and vanilla powder.
- In another bowl (large), combine the eggs with the maple syrup. Add the milk and continue to beat for a few minutes.
- at this point add all the dry ingredients (flour and vanilla) one at a time. Continue stirring for a few minutes.
- Add a little oil or butter to the pan and warm it up.
- Pour a ladle of batter into the pan. Pour it in the center of the pan trying to form a circle.
- Cook on a low heat first on one side and then on the other.

Notes

To optimize your time, you can prepare the batter the night before, and keep it in the fridge. In this case it will become denser but in the morning you will only have to cook the pancakes.

Coconut Crumble With Strawberry And Rhubarb

Ingredients for 3 crumbs

For the stuffing

- 150 grams of strawberries
- 130 grams of rhubarb
- 1 tablespoon of Demerara sugar

- A lemon juice
- Vanilla powder
- 4 tablespoons of water

For the crumble

- 60 grams of small oats
- 60 grams of rice flour
- 25 grams of grated coconut
- 50 grams of extra virgin coconut oil
- 1 tablespoon of maple syrup
- Vanilla powder

Instructions

- Turn on the oven and heat it up to a temperature of 180 ° C.
- Wash the strawberries, then cut them into pieces.
- Wash the rhubarb. Cut it into small pieces.
- Put the rhubarb in a medium-sized saucepan with 4 tablespoons of water, sugar, lemon and vanilla. Cook everything for 10/12 minutes or until the rhubarb is very soft.
- Dissolve coconut oil.
- In a medium-sized bowl mix oats, rice flour, grated coconut, coconut oil, maple syrup and vanilla powder.
- Extinguish the fire. Mix strawberries and rhubarb.
- Divide the fruit into three small baking molds (9 cm) and cover with the mixture of oats, flour and coconut.
- Bake at 180 ° C for 35 minutes.

- Serve with Greek yogurt. You can also use lactose-free yogurt.

Oatmeal Pancake

Ingredients for 5 pancakes or 9 mini-pancakes (2/3 portions)

- 70 gr oatmeal / oatmeal
- 2 eggs
- 180 ml of almond milk
- 1 tablespoon of maple syrup
- Vanilla powder
- Virgin coconut oil or clarified butter

For the seasoning

- Dark chocolate cream
- Fresh fruit (choose the seasonal one)
- Dried fruits (hazelnuts, walnuts, almonds)

Instructions

- In a medium-sized bowl, mix the oatmeal and vanilla powder.
- In another bowl, beat the eggs with maple syrup. Then add the almond milk, continue to beat for a few minutes.
- Add the dry ingredients (oatmeal and vanilla) one at a time. Continue to beat for a few minutes.
- In a pan (preferably non-stick), dissolve the extra virgin coconut or ghee oil, add a ladle of batter and cook for about 4 minutes.

- Turn the pancake over and cook it on the other side for 2 minutes.

Notes

To get a thicker batter, prepare it in advance. If in fact you prepare the night before, leaving it to rest for an entire night in the fridge, the oats will absorb most of the liquid. The batter will become thicker and it will be easier to prepare small pancakes.

Rolled Oats, Brazil Nuts And Dark Chocolate Cookies

Ingredients for 16 biscuits

- 160 grams of gluten-free flour mixture *
- 120 grams of oat flakes (preferably thin and small)
- 50 grams of Brazilian nuts
- 60 grams of dark chocolate
- 90 grams of extra virgin coconut oil
- 80 grams of maple syrup
- 1 egg
- Vanilla powder

Instructions

- Chop the walnuts and Brazilian chocolate (not too small), you can use a knife.
- In a medium-sized bowl, mix the coconut oil (not dissolved) with the maple syrup. Use an electric whisk.
- Add the egg and keep stirring.

- In another medium-sized bowl, place rolled oats and flour. Add the chopped chocolate and nuts. Stir for a few minutes.
- Now place the mixture of oil syrup and the eggs. Keep stirring well.
- Take small portions of pasta with your hands, make small balls flattened. Put them on a baking sheet (with parchment paper) -
- Bake at 190 ° C for 25 minutes.

Notes

* You can use 100 grams of rice flour and 50 grams of potato starch.

The FODMAP content of Brazil nuts is tested by Monash University. 40 grams of Brazilian nuts are LOW-FODMAP results! Brazilian nuts are harvested exclusively in the Amazon rainforest in Bolivia and are not found in other places. They are the only type of dried fruit that is harvested in natural areas without cultivation. They are good and rich in selenium, which is very useful for the immune system.

Carrot Cake

Ingredients for a 24 cm cake pan (10 portions)
- 160 grams of rice flour
- 70 grams of potato starch
- 80 grams of corn starch
- 75 grams of almond flour
- 280 grams of finely grated carrots

- 160 grams of Demerara sugar
- 100 grams of extra virgin coconut oil (or other suitable oil)
- 3 eggs
- 16 grams of baking powder
- 1/2 teaspoon of vanilla powder
- Sliced almonds (to garnish)

Indications

- Dissolve coconut oil. Let it cool for a few minutes
- In a medium-large bowl, combine and mix the flour, ground almonds, baking powder and vanilla.
- Beat the eggs with the sugar until they are soft (use an electric whisk)
- Add melted coconut oil.
- Add the grated carrots and mix well for a few minutes.
- Add dry ingredients.
- Pour the mixture into a cake tin (24 cm) and garnish with sliced almonds.
- Put in a preheated oven at 170 ° C and cook for about 45 minutes.

Buckwheat And Banana Cake

Ingredients

- 70 grams of rice flour
- 70 grams of buckwheat flour
- 2 teaspoons of baking powder

- 1 tablespoon of hazelnut
- 1 tablespoon of almonds
- 1 tablespoon of sunflower seeds
- 100 grams of extra virgin coconut oil, melted
- 1 egg
- 1 banana, crushed
- 2 tablespoons of maple syrup
- 2 tablespoons of coconut yoghurt
- Almond flakes or grated coconut dried to garnish

Instructions

- Chop the nuts and seeds (make them like flour) with a food processor.
- Whisk the egg with the coconut oil and crushed banana. Use an electric mixer.
- Add peanuts, seeds and maple syrup. Continue to beat with the mixer for 1 minute.
- Add the flour, mixed with baking powder and yogurt. Stir very well for another minute.
- Put everything in an oven dish (18 cm) with parchment paper.
- Top with almond flakes or grated coconut
- Cook for about 35 minutes at 170 ° C.

Notes

The banana, buckwheat and extra virgin coconut oil give this cake a delicious taste. A lactose-free, gluten-free and low-sugar cake. The cake is ideal for breakfast or as a snack.

Hot Chocolate With Brazil Nuts

Ingredients for a cup

- 130 ml of almond or rice milk
- 13 grams of dark chocolate (minimum 70%)
- 1 tablespoon of cocoa
- 1 tablespoon of corn starch
- 2 teaspoons of brown sugar or maple syrup (optional)
- vanilla powder
- 2 Brazil nuts, chopped into small pieces

Instructions

- Put the milk in a small pan and heat the milk
- Add the corn starch, cocoa, sugar. Mix well with a spoon. Then use a whisk at the end.
- When the milk is hot (do not boil it), add the chopped chocolate, vanilla powder and sweetener. Continue banging.
- When the milk begins to boil, continue stirring for 2 minutes.
- Serve in a cup with the Brazil nuts on top.

Chapter 5: the low-fodmap diet cookbook for appetizers and main meals

Millet And Chickpeas Falafel

Makes about 12-14 falafel (2 serves)

- 100 gr of millet
- 90 gr of canned chickpeas
- 2 teaspoons of potato starch
- parsley
- the green tops of two spring onions
- half a teaspoon of cumin
- salt
- cooking oil

Directions

- Wash the millet under running water.
- Put the millet in a saucepan and cover it with 250 ml of lightly salted water. Cover with a lid and cook it until the water is completely absorbed.
- Then turn of the heat and let the millet cool slightly.
- Meanwhile, puree the chickpeas using a hand mixer or food processor.
- Chop the parsley and the green tops of spring onions.

- Mix chickpea puree, corn starch, cumin and a pinch of salt. Cool the mixture and set for a while, if it is still too hot.
- Make small balls with small pieces of dough.
- Heat a little oil in the pan and fry the falafels until they turn golden.
- Serve the falafel with yogurt and tahini dressing.

Notes

The portion of chickpeas (strictly canned or in a glass jar) recommended during the elimination phase is 42 grams (per meal), while the double quantity (85 grams) contains high levels of oligosaccharides.

Considering that 40 grams are few to make falafel, part of the chickpeas can be replaced with millet, a cereal that is absolutely LOW-FODMAP and therefore can be consumed without problems.

The result? Very good crispy falafel on the outside and soft on the inside, which have nothing to envy of the originals.

If, during reintroduction, you discover that you can tolerate the galactans contained in legumes, and the fructans contained in garlic and onions, you can certainly go back to the originals, but in the meantime, delight in them.

Savory Cake With Beets, Pumpkin And Feta

Ingredients for about 6 portions

For the crust

- 120 gr of buckwheat flour
- 50 gr of rice flour

- 50 gr of potato starch*
- 1 egg
- 50 gr of extra-virgin olive oil
- 50 ml of water

For the filling

- 200/250 gr of raw pumpkin (peeled and deseeded)
- 100 gr of beets
- 2 eggs
- 200 ml of unsweetened almond milk
- 150 gr of feta
- Green tops of two spring onions
- Fresh parsley
- Salt
- Pepper
- Any kind of oil (suitable for cooking)

Directions

- Preheat the oven to 190°C.
- Cut the pumpkin into rather small chunks, Put them on a baking tray covered with parchment paper, season them with oil and salt. Cook it in the oven for about 15 minutes or until it's fork-tender.
- In a bowl combine the ingredients and make a soft dough. Allow the mixture to cool.
- Make small balls with small pieces of dough.
- Fry the falafels in the pan until they turn golden.

- Serve the falafel with my yogurt and tahini dressing.
- In the meanwhile, prepare the crust: in a bowl put the buckwheat flour, rice flour and potato starch, the egg (beaten), extra-virgin olive oil and salt.
- Mix the ingredients with a fork and then with your fingers until they are well combined, then start adding the water and keep mixing the ingredients with your hands. The result should be a nice ball of pastry.
- At this point, beets and pumpkin should be ready. Turn off the heat and take the pumpkin out of the oven. Lower the temperature to 170°C.
- Grease a quiche pan of 24 cm with a removable bottom. Roll out the dough directly into the pan. Prick the pastry with a fork, place a baking sheet on the crust and add something heavy and dry (beans, uncooked grains) to blink-bake it for 12 minutes.
- Meanwhile, in a bowl whisk two eggs, add the almond milk and the crumbled feta. Season with salt, pepper, and fresh parsley. Add the cooked and cooled beets.
- When the crust is ready, add on top of it three-quarters of the cooked pumpkin. Then pour the eggs, feta and beets mixture. Finally, add the last pieces of pumpkin.
- Cook the quiche in the oven at 175°C for about 45-50 minutes.

Note

*Potato starch makes the crust a bit more crunchy. If you prefer a more chewy dough, you can replace the starch with 40 gr of oat flour.

Endive Soup

Ingredients for 2 serves

- 180 gr of endive (the green one)
- 200 gr of potatoes
- The green top of one spring onion
- 450 ml of stock or water*
- 2 tablespoon of pine nuts
- 2 sun-dried tomatoes
- 2 tablespoons of Parmesan
- 2 tablespoons of extra-virgin olive oil
- Salt
- Pepper

Directions

- Clean and cut the endive and the potatoes into chunks.
- Heat 2 tablespoons in a rather big pot and add the green top of spring onion.
- Add the endive and 200 grams (two thirds) of the potatoes, salt and pepper.
- Add the broth, put a lid and cook the veggies at medium-low heat for about 30 minutes, or until they are soft.
- In the meanwhile, you can steam the remaining potato chunks and put them aside.

- Turn off the heat and blend the vegetables using an hand blender.
- Add the parmesan and stir. Then you can put the pan again on the stove and cook for 10 more minutes on medium heat, if you want to make the soup nice and thick.
- In a small pan, toast the pine nuts. Be careful not to burn them!
- Cut the sun-dried tomatoes into small pieces.
- Serve the endive soup, topped with the steamed potatoes, sun-dried tomatoes and pine nuts.

Notes

* I used chicken bone broth, which has incredible healing properties, but you can also use vegetable stock or water.

This escarole cream is easy to prepare, is made with ingredients available in all supermarkets, and is ideal as a first course, especially in winter. Despite being a simple dish, this velvety is really tasty: the slightly bitter taste of the escarole is balanced by the more neutral flavor of the potatoes. The dried tomatoes and pine nuts give the final touch!

Be careful because the dried tomatoes are to be consumed in moderation: if two dry tomatoes (7 grams) are LOW-FODMAP, 4 tomatoes (15 grams) already contain moderate amounts of fructose. However they are so rich in taste.

Moreover, since all the other ingredients are allowed without particular restrictions, this recipe can certainly be considered LOW-FODMAP.

Slow Cooked - Beef Stew

Ingredients

- 350 grams of braising beef (I use grass-fed)
- 150 grams of carrots
- 150 grams of potatoes
- 10 grams of celery
- 3tablespoons of tomato puree
- 250 ml of broth (any kind, preferably homemade)
- Corn starch (potato starch or tapioca)
- 1-2 leaves of laurel
- Chives or green tops of spring onions
- Thyme. q.b.
- Salt
- Pepper
- Ghee (clarified butter) or any kind of fat

Directions

- Wash, peel and cut the vegetables into chunks, put them in the slow cooker.
- Pat dry the meat with some kitchen paper, cut it into chunks and cover them with corn starch (or tapioca or potato starch).
- In a non-stick pan, heat some ghee (or any other fat) and brown the meat on medium-high heat. Transfer it into the slow cooker.

- Pour the broth and the tomato puree into the pan in which you have browned the meat and stir for about one minute. Pour the liquid into the crockpot.
- Add salt, pepper and herbs (thyme, laurel, chives) and stir so that everything is well mixed.
- Cook with the lid on and low for about 5 hours. When this time has passed, remove the lid, give it a good stir and if you prefer a more dry stew, then cook on high for about half an hour (up to one hour) without the lid.

Quinoa With Vegetables And Lemon Scent

Makes 2-3 serves

- 150 (black) quinoa
- 200 gr of cod (2 fillets)
- 200 gr of mixed veggies
- 1 tablespoon of ground cumin
- 1 tablespoon of oregano
- 1/2 tablespoon of ground coriander
- Chili pepper, to taste (optional)
- Parsley
- Chives
- Salt
- Lemon juice
- Extra-virgin olive oil
- Extra-virgin coconut oil (or other suitable cooking oil)

Directions

- Place the quinoa in a colander, wash it and cook it according to the instructions on the package.
- In a bowl mix cumin, oregano, coriander, chili pepper, parsley, and half tablespoon of salt.
- Mix three quarter of the mixture together with one tablespoon of olive oil and one of lemon juice.
- Put the fillets in a baking pan adding the mixture of oil, lemon and spices. Let them marinate for 20 minutes.
- In the meanwhile, wash the veggies and chop them into small pieces. Heat one tablespoon of extra-virgin coconut oil in a non-stick pan, add chives the veggies and let them brown. Then add the remaining spices mixture, a bit of water (so they don't get too dry), cover and cook until tender.
- Cook the fish fillets in the upper part of a preheated oven at 200° for about 25 minutes.
- Add the quinoa to the veggies and give them a good stir. Add a bit more salt, if desired. Divide the quinoa-veggies mix into plates
- When the fish is cooked, then shred the fillets using a fork. Put some on top of the quinoa, add some cooking juice and a splash of lemon juice. You can also stir everything together, quinoa, veggies and shredded cod fillets along with their juice.

Notes

Quinoa is a pseudo-cereal that belongs to the same family as spinach and beetroot. However, given the high concentration of starchy carbohydrates, quinoa has a nutritional profile similar to that of the cereals we normally use for our first courses.

Unlike pasta and rice, however, quinoa contains a greater quantity of proteins and unsaturated fats, a lower glycemic load and a greater satiety index.

Like rice, buckwheat and amaranth and corn, quinoa is gluten-free, so it is also suitable for those with celiac disease.

Quinoa is suitable for all those who follow the LOW-FODMAP diet, however, due to the high fiber content, some people with IBS may have some complaints.

The advice therefore is to eat half a portion at first and see how it goes.

The Veggie Tartare With Lemon Juice

Ingredients for 2/3 servings

- 60 gr of avocado
- 150 gr of zucchini
- 130 grams of deseeded cucumber
- Lemon juice
- Extra-virgin olive oil
- Pepper
- Fresh herbs (parsley, basil, chives, mint)

Instructions

- Cut the vegetables and the avocado into small pieces.
- Put them in a bowl and add salt, pepper, lemon juice, olive oil and chopped herbs.

- Mix well for a few minutes.
- Divide the mixture into 3-4 greased molds and arrange the mixture using a spoon.
- Put the molds in the refrigerator for 40 minutes and then turn them on a plate.
- Offer the tartare with toasted gluten-free bread or some rocket.

Notes

Fresh and light recipe: veggie tartare!

Perfect as an appetizer or side dish during a summer dinner.

Omelette With Sweet Potato, Spinach And Feta

Makes 2 portions

- 4 eggs
- 150 grams (1 large) sweet potatoes, washed and peeled*
- 75 grams (2 cups) of fresh spinach, washed
- 75 grams (2,5 ounces) of feta
- Thyme
- Salt
- Pepper
- Extra-virgin olive oil

Instructions

- Preheat the oven at 200° C.
- Snip the sweet potatoes into thin slices (not cubes) and steam them.

- Meanwhile, in a frying pan heat a teaspoon of oil and quickly sauté the spinach. Put them aside.
- In a bowl, crumble the feta using the back of a fork, then add eggs and whisk everything together. Add a bit of salt, pepper, thyme and finally the cooked spinach.
- With the same pan in which you cooked the spinach, heat about two teaspoons of oil, then add the chives and finally the sweet potatoes. Roast them on both sides until they are beautifully golden and season with salt and pepper.
- Set them on a baking dish (20x20) covered with parchment paper.
- Pour the egg, feta and spinach mixture over the potatoes.
- Bake the omelette in a preheated oven for about 20 minutes or until the top starts to brown.

Notes

* Up to 70 gr of sweet potato is LOW- FODMAP, therefore you should able to eat approximately half of this omelette (1 portion) without any issue.

Brown Rice Spaghetti With Black Cabbage

Makes 4

- 330 grams of brown rice spaghetti

For the pesto

- 100 grams of black cabbage
- 2 heaped tablespoons of pine nuts
- 4 tablespoons extra-virgin olive oil

- A splash of lemon juice
- Salt
- Pepper
- 2 tablespoons toasted pine nuts to garnish

Instructions

- Wash the black cabbage and cut it into pieces.
- Steam it for about 20 minutes and let it cool.
- Meanwhile bring the water to boil (to cook the pasta).
- In a blender, put the black cabbage leaves, pine nuts, olive oil, lemon juice, salt, pepper and blend everything until smooth.
- Set some salt in the water, add the pasta and cook it according to the instructions on the package.
- Meanwhile, transfer the pesto in a large bowl and add 4 tablespoons of the cooking water, stir well.
- When the pasta is ready, add pesto and put it in the bowl.
- Mix well and divide into two bowls and then top it with toasted pine nuts.

Notes

Please note immediately that the black cabbage has unfortunately not yet been tested (also because in Australia perhaps they do not even know what it is), so it is better to consume it in moderation.

Vegan Lentil Burgers

Makes 4

- 230 grams canned lentil, well rinsed and drained
- 1 medium carrot (70gr), grated
- 40 grams fine oats
- 2 tablespoons extra virgin olive oil
- 1 tablespoon of chives
- Parsley
- Salt
- Pepper
- Cooking oil or ghee

Instructions

- Place all the ingredients (except the cooking oil) in a food processor and process until you get a nice compact mixture and everything is well-mixed.*
- Form the mixture into four patties.**
- In a pan, heat 2 tablespoons of cooking oil and cook the burgers on both sides. Cook until they are golden brown.

Notes

* You can certainly add spices, such as cumin, turmeric or garam masala.

** Don't worry if the mixture looks too soft: it will become more firm while cooking. However, if it is impossible to shape it into patties, then you can add more oats or let the mixture rest in the refrigerator for at least one hour, so that it becomes more compact.

Polenta Wedges With Red Endive

Makes 6

- 280 gr of polenta
- 1 liter of vegetable stock (or water)
- 650 gr of red Belgian endive (or radicchio)
- Pecorino cheese, flaked
- Clarified butter (ghee) or extra-virgin olive oil
- Chives
- Parsley
- Salt
- Pepper

Instructions

- Boil the vegetable stock, add some salt and turn off the heat.
- Pour the polenta slowly in the stock while stirring with a whisk.
- Turn on the heat and cook the polenta over low heat for about 10 minutes while continuing to stir with a whisk in order to make no lumps.
- Pour the polenta into a non-stick baking dish (eventually made of glass) of about 30x20 cm and let it cool.
- Meanwhile, wash and thinly cut the red endive (or radicchio).

- Melt a bit of ghee (or olive oil) in a non-stick pan, add chives and then endive (or chicory).
- Add salt, pepper and parsley.
- Then low the heat and cover with a lid. Let it simmer for about 10 minutes.
- Remove the lid and continue cooking the endive (or radicchio) for about 5 minutes, until it becomes a bit more dry.
- Put the polenta on a cutting board and using a small bowl (diameter 10 cm) make some round-shaped wedges.
- In a pan heat a bit more ghee (or extra-virgin olive oil) and roast the polenta wedges on both sides until they are nice and gold.
- Arrange them on a plate and garnish with endive (or radicchio), Pecorino flakes, and a bit of pepper or a drizzle of extra virgin olive oil to taste.

Notes

If you want to make a vegan version of this recipe, you can replace the pecorino with walnuts or flaked almonds. For a "carnivorous" version, you can instead add a little speck or bacon.

Orange And Thyme Chicken

Ingredients for 2 servings
- 450-500 gr organic or free-range chicken (thighs with bone)
- 120 ml of fresh orange juice
- Thyme

- Parsley
- Chives (optional)
- Salt
- Pepper
- Ghee

Instructions:

- Spread some butter in the bottom of the pan.
- Add salt to the chicken and place it in the slow cooker.
- Rub the chicken skin with ghee (you can skip this passage, if you prefer).
- Pour the orange juice over the chicken.
- Add herbs, salt and pepper.
- Cook on low for 6 hours.

Zucchini Crusted With Fillets Of Plaice

Ingredients for 2 servings

- 280 grams Fillets of plaice
- 1 zucchini
- Almond meal (or white ground almonds)
- Extra virgin olive oil
- Chives (optional)
- Parsley
- Lemon
- Salt
- Pepper

Instructions

- Put the plaice fillets in a greased oven-proof dish.
- Marinate the fillets with a splash of lemon juice and a pinch of salt.
- Meanwhile, finely cut the zucchini into rounds.
- Then place the zucchini on plaice fillets.
- Using a pastry brush, evenly spread EVO oil on zucchini.
- Sprinkle with almond flour.
- Season with a bit of salt, pepper, chives and parsley.
- Bake in preheated oven (180°C) for about 12 minutes (grill, possibly), placing the dish on one of the highest level.

Notes

This recipe is a light and tasty dish, it is prepared in no time, and is perfect for a midweek dinner.

Instead of plaice, you can use any other type of white fish (cod, sole, sea bass ...). I advise you not to use frozen fish because when cooking in the oven it would release a lot of water and make the dish less appetizing.

Millet Croquettes With Zucchini And Basil

Ingredients (1 serve)

- 75 grams millet
- 70 grams zucchini, grated
- 1-2 teaspoons of corn starch (or potato starch or tapioca)
- 20 grams of Parmesan, grated

- Basil (2 leaves)
- Salt
- Pepper
- Chives
- (Extra-virgin) coconut oil

Instructions

- Cook the millet. You can following the instructions on the packet.
- Heat a bit of oil in a pan, add chives, zucchini, salt, pepper and cook for about 5 minutes.
- Let the millet and the zucchini to cool.
- In a bowl, mix the cooked millet, corn starch, parmesan, pumpkin, salt, pepper, sage (chopped).
- Form small-medium balls*.
- Cook in a pan with a bit of coconut oil until golden brown.

Notes

*If the mixture crumbles, put it in the fridge in order to make it more firm.

Oven-Baked Salmon With Dill

Ingredients for 2 serves

- 2 fillets of fresh salmon (about 140 grams each)
- Lemon juice
- Salt

- Pepper
- Dill
- 1 zucchini (100 gr.)
- Chives
- Extra-virgin olive oil
- Ghee

Instructions

- Preheat oven 200°C (ventilated, grill).
- Put the salmon in a greased pan
- Pour the lemon juice on the salmon fillets, add a bit of extra virgin olive oil, salt, pepper and dill. Let it marinate for 15 minutes.
- Meanwhile, wash zucchini and "spiralize" them using the spiralizer.
- Place the salmon in the oven. Cook for 15 minutes.
- Warm up a bit of ghee in a pan, add chives, zucchini, a bit of salt and pepper.
- Cook for about 10 minutes. You can cook until the zucchini noodles are soft.
- Offer immediately the salmon and zucchini noodle as a side.

Notes

To make zucchini spaghetti, you need an object called "spiralizer". This tool is becoming very popular among food bloggers, above all because it allows to obtain perfect vegetable and gluten-free noodles, made with zucchini, carrots, but also potatoes or other vegetables.

If you can't find the coiling machine, you can use a potato peeler or a mandolin and make zucchini noodles instead of spaghetti.

Zucchini are LOW-FODMAP, but be careful because portions over 100g. they contain high amounts of Oligosaccharides (fructans).

Finally, for this recipe, try to find fresh and good quality salmon: the frozen one is really something else!

Beef Burger With Eggplant Bun

Ingredients for 4 burgers

- 500 grams ground beef (grass-fed or organic)
- 3-4 teaspoons chives
- 1/2 teaspoon paprika
- 1/2 teaspoon ground coriander
- 1/2 teaspoon ground ginger
- 1/2 teaspoon parsley
- 1/4 teaspoon chili
- Salt (to taste)
- Ghee
- 2 eggplant slices

Instructions

- First of all, mix all the herbs, spices and salt.
- Add this mixture to minced meat, mix quickly and set aside.
- Meanwhile, cook the eggplant: heat a grill and put on the eggplant slices. Cook until they are tender.

- Shape the meat into 4 round balls and flatten them.
- In a large skillet warm 1/2 teaspoon of ghee.
- Cook burgers for about 8-10 minutes (depends how you like them). Flip them when they are half-cooked.
- Place the burger between the eggplant slices. Garnish as desired.

Vegetable Curry

Ingredients (2 serves)

- 450 grams mixed vegetables: 220 grams of starchy veggies, such as parsnips, potatoes or sweet potatoes* + 320 grams of regular veggies, such as broccoli, carrots, zucchini or eggplants
- 220 ml. full-fat coconut milk
- 1 tablespoon of coconut oil
- 1 teaspoon chives
- 1/2 teaspoon cumin
- 1/2 teaspoon turmeric
- 1/4 teaspoon coriander
- 1/4 teaspoon ground ginger
- 1/4 teaspoon paprika
- A pinch of cinnamon
- A pinch of chili pepper
- A pinch of salt

Instructions

- Cut, and then clean, the vegetables into small pieces.
- Steam the veggies for 13/15 minutes.
- Mix the spices in a container.
- Heat a tablespoon of extra virgin coconut in a pan.
- Add the chives, the mix of spices and then vegetables and salt. Let it brown.
- Add the coconut milk and cook over low heat for 15 minutes more or less.

Notes

*Less than 75 grams/serve.

This is the recipe for a LOW-FODMAP dish, vegan, paleo and at the same time nutritious and tasty. "Impossible", you might think, and instead it is possible: this vegetable-based curry is really tasty, satiating and healthy, though not containing onion or garlic, foods of animal origin, cereals or legumes. In addition, coconut milk and starchy vegetables, such as sweet potato and parsnip, make this dish much more nutritious than a simple side dish.

To make this curry, you can use the vegetables you like the most depending on seasonal availability, but the advice is to also include starchy vegetables, such as sweet potatoes, in order to make it more substantial.

Quinoa And Spinach Croquettes

Ingredients (2 serves)
- 150 grams quinoa
- 40 grams Parmesan, grated

- 200 grams of fresh spinach
- Salt
- Pepper
- Thyme
- Chives
- Parsley
- Extra virgin coconut oil or sunflower seeds oil

Instructions

- Cook the quinoa according to the instructions on the package.
- In a frying pan, add a little olive oil to warm, add the chives and spinach. Cook for 12-15 minutes with the lid.
- Place cooked quinoa, cooked spinach, grated Parmesan, salt, pepper, thyme and parsley in a blender and blend until well combined. If your blender is too small, blend the quinoa first, then spinach and, in a bowl, mix everything using your hands, after you have added salt, pepper, thyme and parsley.
- Take small portions of the mixture and shape them into small balls.
- Place some oil in a pan and cook the croquettes for about 5 minutes until brown.

Notes

As far as spinach is concerned, they too are LOW-FODMAP like quinoa, but portions of 150 grams must not be exceeded. because they contain moderate amounts of oligo-fructans and are therefore to be avoided.

Dukkah-Crusted Cod Fillets

Ingredients (4 serves)

- 4 cod fillets (about 150g. each one)
- 2 tbsp extra-virgin olive oil
- A splash of lemon juice
- A pinch of salt
- Pepper

For the Dukkah

- 2 tablespoons peeled hazelnuts
- 2 tablespoons sesame
- 2 teaspoons of chia seeds (or black sesame)
- 1 teaspoon cumin
- A pinch of salt

Instructions

- Marinate the cod fillets in lemon juice, salt and pepper.
- Meanwhile, roughly chop the hazelnuts (using an electric mixer), pour them on a baking tray and put it in the oven at 220 degrees for about 10 minutes (grill), until lightly brown. Be careful not to burn them!
- Roast in a pan the sesame seeds in until they start popping.
- Mix hazelnuts, sesame seeds, chia seeds, cumin and salt. Put this mixture into a plate.
- Pour two tablespoon of extra-virgin olive oil into a bowl.

- Dip one side of the cod fillets first in the oil and then coat them with the Dukkah (mixture of hazelnuts, sesame and cumin).
- Put the cod fillets down on a baking tray greased with the remaining oil and bake in preheated oven at 200°C for 13/15 minutes (grill function).

Notes

Dukkah is an Egyptian blend of spices, nuts and seeds. Traditionally it is consumed by dipping a piece of bread, previously dipped in olive oil. Otherwise, it can be mixed with salads or vegetables, or it is used to "bread" meat or fish, so as to form a crunchy and tasty crust.

Turmeric And Poppy Seeds Chicken And Veggies

Ingredients (2 serves)

- 320 gr chicken breast (organic)
- 320 gr mixed seasonal vegetables (carrots, broccoli, pumpkin, zucchini, eggplant ...)
- 3 level tablespoons of tapioca (or rice flour or potato starch)
- 1 teaspoon turmeric
- 1 teaspoon poppy seeds (optional)
- 2 tablespoons of coconut oil
- Salt
- Pepper
- Chives

- Herbs to taste (parsley, coriander)

Instructions

- Clean, chop and steam the vegetables.
- Snip the chicken breast into small pieces.
- In a bowl, mix the flour, a pinch of salt and turmeric.
- Coat the chicken pieces with the mixture of flour, salt and turmeric.
- Put a spoonful of coconut oil in a pan and heat. Then add the chicken.
- Let them cook for about 6 minutes.
- Place the chicken in a plate.
- Put in another tablespoon of coconut oil in the same pan used for chicken.
- Put in the vegetables, a pinch of salt and stir-fry the veggies for about 1-2 minutes.
- Add the chicken, poppy seeds and finally pepper and herbs to taste.

Notes

A quick and simple recipe: nothing special, but that can give an extra idea for a midweek lunch or dinner. In fact, when you start following this diet, you often run out of ideas. Your diet is limited to very few foods and you are often persecuted by the sense of hunger.

Zucchini And Bacon Muffin

Ingredients for 12-13 muffins

- 85 grams rice flour
- 35 grams corn starch
- 2 teaspoons of baking powder
- 5 eggs
- 250 grams zucchini, grated
- 100 grams hard cheese, grated (such as Parmesan, Pecorino, Gouda...)
- 85 grams bacon, chopped
- 2 tablespoons of extra-virgin olive oil
- Parsley
- Chives (optional)
- A pinch of salt
- Ghee

Instructions

- Beat the eggs.
- Put in the flour, starch and baking powder, sifted.
- Add the other ingredients and mix well.
- Pour the mixture in a greased (with ghee) and floured muffin tin.
- Cook for 30 minutes 180°C.

Notes

You can replace bacon with small pieces of carrots, red pepper or sun-dried tomatoes, if you prefer a vegetarian version.

Carrots And Turmeric Velvety Soup

Ingredients (2 serves)

- 200 grams (1 cup) of potato
- 120 grams (1/2 cup) of pumpkin
- 80 grams (1/3 cup) of carrot
- 500 ml (2 cups) of vegetable stock
- 1/2 teaspoon of turmeric
- Chives
- Coriander leaves (fresh or dried)
- Extra-virgin coconut oil (or ghee)
- Salt
- Pepper
- Poppy, sunflower or pumpkin seeds to garnish
- 3-5 tablespoons of coconut milk

Instructions

• Clean and cut the vegetables into small pieces.

• Heat a bit of coconut oil/ghee in a pan and add the chives.

• Add all the vegetables, turmeric, coriander, salt and pepper.

• Cover with the stock and cook for about 30 minutes, or until the vegetables are soft.

• Finish cooking and cool for at least 5 minutes.

• Puree the vegetables using an hand blender.

• Put in the coconut milk and keep blending.

- Adorn with poppy seeds (or pumpkin seeds, if you prefer) and serve with a slice of spelt bread (sourdough), toasted.

Notes

After having blended the vegetables, you can put the pan again on the heat to make the soup thicker.

Chapter 6: the low-fodmap diet cookbook for side dishes

Parsnip And Turmeric Cous Cous

Makes 5-6 serves

- 500 gr of parsnip
- fresh turmeric*
- Oil suitable for cooking (or ghee)
- chives or tree tops of spring onions
- salt
- pepper
- fresh parsley

Directions

- Remove the peel of the parsnips and cut them into big chunks.
- Put the parsnip chunks into a big and powerful food processor. Pulse them until they reach the size of rice or cuscus.
- Peel and grate a small piece of fresh turmeric.
- Het a couple of tablespoons of oil (or one tablespoon of ghee) and add one teaspoon turmeric.
- Add the parsnip cous cous, the chives (or tree tops of spring onions) and stir so that the cuscus becomes nice and yellow.
- Put in salt and pepper, cover with a lid and let it cook for about 15 minutes on low heat.

- When it is cooked, add the fresh parsley.
- You can use the parsnip cous cous as a side to soak up the liquid of a stew or with my turmeric chicken.

Notes

*You can replace the fresh turmeric with one teaspoon of turmeric powder.

Kale Chips

Makes 1-2 servings

- 85 gr of kale, washed
- 2 level tablespoons of extra-virgin olive oil
- Salt to taste

Instructions

- Preheat the oven at 160°C.
- Remove the cabbage leaves from the stems and wash it. Calculate 70 grams of leaves without stems.
- Place the kale in a bowl, add a bit of salt and two level tablespoons of extra-virgin oil.
- Use your hands to start massaging the kale well so that all the leaves are totally covered with the oil.
- Cook the cabbage (put on baking paper) in the oven for 17/20 minutes. You can cook until the leaves begin to brown.

Notes

Do not overdo with the oil otherwise the leaves may soften too much.

It is absolutely necessary that the leaves are well spread on the baking sheet and that they do not overlap, otherwise they might not cook properly or become soggy.

Braised Red Cabbage

Ingredients for about 6-8 portions

- 1/2 red cabbage (about 700 gr.)
- 2 tablespoons raisins
- 1 cup (250ml) of water or vegetable stock
- Chives
- 2 tablespoons of apple cider vinegar
- Salt
- Pepper
- Clarified butter (ghee)

Instructions

- Wash and finely cut the cabbage.
- Heat a little butter in the pan.
- Add chives and cabbage.
- Pour two tablespoons of apple cider vinegar on the cabbage cooking on high heat and let it evaporate.
- Add salt, pepper, vegetable stock and cover with a lid.
- Let the cabbage cook over low heat for about 40 minutes. If you see that it gets too dry, add a little bit of hot water.
- After 15 minutes, you can add the raisins. Stir and cook with the lid until cooked.

Italian Mashed Potatoes

Ingredients (2 serves)

- 300 grams of starchy potatoes
- 150 ml of lactose-free milk
- 2 tablespoons of grated Parmesan
- 1/2 teaspoon of ghee (or clarified butter)
- Salt
- Pepper or nutmeg to taste

Instructions

- Steam the potatoes.
- Mash the potatoes with a potato masher.
- In a saucepan, pour the milk and heat it on low heat.
- Add the mashed potatoes and stir.
- Put in the Parmesan cheese, salt, pepper or nutmeg and finally the butter.
- Stir to obtain a creamy and smooth potato puree.

No-Fried Chips With Thyme-Scented

Ingredients (2 serves)

- 250 gr potatoes
- 1 tablespoon of extra virgin olive oil
- Thyme
- Salt and pepper

Instructions

- Snip the potatoes into sticks and place on a baking tray covered with parchment paper.
- In a small cup mix the oil with thyme, salt and pepper.
- Brush the potatoes with the herbed oil.
- Bake the potatoes in the upper part of the oven for about 25-30 minutes at 200° C.

Fennel And Orange Salad

Ingredients (2 serves)

- 100 grams fennel
- 1 orange
- Any kind of seed (poppy seeds, chia seeds)
- 2 tablespoons extra-virgin olive oil
- Salt
- Pepper

Instructions

- Wash the fennel and chop it thinly.
- Peel the orange and slice it thinly.
- In a bowl combine the oil, salt and pepper.
- Add fennel, orange and mix well.
- Add a sprinkle of seeds to taste.

Notes

You can replace the seeds, with any other kind of nuts, with toasted pine nuts for instance.

Chapter 7: the low-fodmap diet cookbook for snack e smoothie

Gianduia Cream

Ingredients for two nice-creams

- 2 medium ripe bananas
- 2 teaspoons of hazelnut butter*
- 3 teaspoons of cacao
- Ten roasted hazelnuts
- 1-2 tablespoons of vegetable milk

Instructions

- Cut the peeled bananas into slices. Put them in a freezer bag for at least 4 hours, or even longer.
- Place the frozen and sliced bananas in a powerful blender along with the other ingredients (except whole hazelnuts).
- Blend until everything is nice and creamy. You may have to scrape the ice-cream from time to time, if it sticks to the edges of the food processor.
- Stir in the whole hazelnuts and divide the cream into two bowls.

Sunflower Crackers With Sun-Dried Tomatoes And Oregano

Ingredients for about 22-25 crackers

- 120 gr sunflower seeds
- 85 gr almond flour (or ground white almonds)
- 25 gr sun-dried tomatoes, well drained
- 1 large egg
- oregano
- salt

Instructions

- Grind the sunflower seeds using a food processor.
- Add sun-dried tomatoes and blend.
- Place the almond meal in a bowl and add the mixture of seeds and sun-dried tomatoes.
- Put in the egg, salt, oregano and mix well. The consistency should be a bit sticky, but not too much.
- Put the dough on a sheet of waxed paper. Cover the dough with another sheet of paper and roll out using a rolling pin.
- Using a sharp knife, cut out little squares.
- Put in the oven and cook at 170/180 ° C for 20/25 minutes.

Matcha And Kiwi Smoothie

Ingredients for 2 smoothies

- 2 kiwi, ripe
- 1 teaspoons of matcha powder
- 1 banana, ripe
- 280 ml (1/4 cup) almond milk (unsweetened)

Instructions

- Snip the banana into small pieces, put it in a freezer bag and store it in the freezer for at least 3,5 hours (overnight would be perfect).
- After this time, place all the ingredients in a powerful blender or food processor.
- Blend until creamy.
- Offer immediately.

Chapter 8: the low-fodmap diet cookbook for sauces and condiments

Spinach Pesto

Ingredients to fill a small jar of pesto (3 portions)

- 45 grams of fresh spinach (or baby spinach), washed and dried
- 25 grams of white almonds
- 30-40 grams of Parmesan
- 2-3 tablespoons of extra virgin olive oil

Instructions

- Place all the dry ingredients (spinach, almonds, parmesan) in a food processor.
- Blend until everything is well-mixed.
- Add 2 tablespoons of olive oil, continue blending until creamy.

- If you decide not to eat the pesto immediately, put it in a small jar and cover it with a tablespoon of extra virgin olive oil. Keep refrigerated.

Notes

You can spread this pesto on bread or use it as a pasta dressing. If so, I suggest you put it first in a bowl (while the pasta is cooking) and dilute it with two tablespoons of the pasta cooking water. Finally, drain the pasta and mix it with pesto.

Basil Pesto

Ingredients (2 servings)

- 20 grams of fresh basil
- 40 grams Parmigiano Reggiano
- 2 tablespoons pine nuts
- 4 tablespoons of (garlic infused) extra virgin olive oil

Instructions

- Wash the basil leaves and dry them gently with a rag.
- Now, you can place all the ingredients in a blender and blend them until you have a homogeneous mixture.
- Add the oil and keep blending until creamy.

Notes

If you decide to use the pesto as a pasta dressing, I suggest you to dilute it by adding two tablespoons of water from the cooking pasta.

Winter Pesto

Ingredients for 2-3 serves

- 100 grams broccoli (only the tops)
- 40 grams Parmesan
- 2 tablespoons pine nuts
- 2 heaped tablespoons of (garlic-infused) extra-virgin olive oil
- A pinch of salt
- Pepper (optional)

Instructions

- Steam the broccoli. Let them cool for 6 minutes.
- Put parmesan, pine nuts, broccoli, salt and pepper in a blender. Blend until creamy.
- Finally, add the olive oil and blend 30 seconds more.

Notes

You can use the pesto as a (gluten-free) pasta sauce or as a dip to spread on (gluten-free) toast. If you decide to use it as a pasta sauce, I suggest you dilute it with 3 tablespoons of the pasta cooking water.

Vanilla Dark Chocolate Spread

Ingredients

- 100 grams of hazelnut butter *
- 50 grams dark chocolate (min. 70%)
- 2 teaspoons of cocoa
- 1 tablespoon extra-virgin coconut oil
- Vanilla powder

Instructions

- First, dissolve the coconut oil and chocolate in a double boiler.
- Put all the ingredients in a blender until creamy.
- If you prefer a more solid consistency, let it rest in the fridge for 3 hours.

Notes

* With a powerful blender, you can make your own homemade hazelnut butter toasting the hazelnuts (for about 12 minutes 175°C) and blending them until creamy.

**You can replace the coconut oil with any other type of oil. In this case, however, it won't be necessary to melt it together with the chocolate.

Raspberry Jam And Chia Seeds

Ingredients

- 180 gr of raspberries
- 1 tablespoon of chia seeds (about 12 gr)
- 2 teaspoons of Demerara sugar (or other sweetener to choice)
- 4 tablespoons (30 ml) of water
- A few drops of lemon juice

Directions

- Wash the raspberries with cold water.
- Place the raspberries in a saucepan together with water, sugar, a few drops of lemon juice.

- Cook about 16 minutes over low heat.
- Finish cooking, add chia seeds.
- Place the jam in a jar, let it cool and put in the fridge for about 6 hours (the chia seeds will absorb the remaining liquid, making the jam nice and jelly.

Yogurt With Tahini

Makes 2

- 2 tablespoons of lactose-free yogurt
- 1 tablespoon of tahini
- Few drops of lemon juice
- a pinch of cumin

Instructions

- Just mix all the ingredients.

Notes

You can prepare your tahini by toasting the sesame seeds in a pan (in the oven, preheated before at 180 ° C for about 12 minutes) until golden brown, then processing them until they are soft and creamy.

FODMAP tip: 1 tablespoon (20 grams) of tahini is LOW-FODMAP. Larger quantities (2 tablespoons, 40 grams), for example, contain high amounts of oligo-fructans.

Chapter 9: the low-fodmap diet cookbook for desserts

Macadamia Nuts Cheesecake With Blueberries

Makes a small cake (18 cm), 12 portions

For the base

- 120 gr of pecans
- 50 gr of almond flour
- 20 gr of extra-virgin coconut oil (melted)
- 20 gr of maple syrup

For the middle layer

- 220 gr of macadamia nuts
- A can (350 ml) of coconut milk
- 60 ml of lemon (or lime) juice
- 4 tablespoons of maple syrup
- 1/2 teaspoon vanilla powder
- For the top layer
- 280 gr of blueberries
- Half a glass of water
- 1 tablespoon of maple syrup (optional)
- A splash of lemon juice
- Vanilla powder, to taste

Instructions

- The night before, put the macadamia nuts in a bowl, and cover them with warm water. Leave them to soak overnight (or at least for 6-8 hours). Also place the coconut milk tin in the refrigerator, so that the fatty part separates from the more liquid part.
- In order to make the base, the following day, cover the bottom of a removable bottom pan with parchment paper. It is important that the pan is of the right dimensions, that is 18 cm.
- Blend pecans in a food processor until they become fine flour. But don't process them too much otherwise you'll get pecan butter instead of flour.
- In a bowl, combine the pecan flour along with the almond flour, the extra virgin coconut oil (melted) and the maple syrup. Mix well and put the mixture into the cake pan, pressing with the back of a spoon to make base for the cake evenly spread. Put the base in the refrigerator to set.
- Meanwhile prepare the middle layer: in a large blender put the macadamia nuts previously soaked and drained well. Then open the coconut milk can and remove the solid part only, which should be now on the surface (you can use the liquid part to make other recipes, such as smoothies). Combine the coconut cream with the macadamia nuts.
- Then add the other ingredients: lemon juice, vanilla powder and maple syrup.
- Blend everything until the mixture reaches a creamy consistency. Pour the mixture over the base; and put everything in the freezer for at least an hour to set.

- Meanwhile prepare the top layer: in a saucepan pour the well washed blueberries, add half cup of water, lemon juice, vanilla and maple syrup. Cook over low heat until the blueberry compote thickens (about 40 minutes). Let it cool completely and then pour on the cake.
- Place the cake in the freezer. I suggest you remove it from the freezer half an hour before serving.

Notes

You can also cut the cake into slices, keep them in the freezer and eat one when you crave something sweet. Just remember to remove it from the freezer about half an hour before eating it.

Vegan Chocolate Tart

Ingredients for 6-8 servings

For the crust

- 130 gr of porridge oats
- 100 gr of hazelnuts
- 50 gr of maple syrup
- For the filling
- 400 ml of full fat coconut milk (canned)
- 90 gr of dark chocolate (min. 70%)
- 2 tablespoons of maple syrup
- 2 tablespoons of tapioca
- Vanilla powder

Instructions

- Preheat the oven 180°C.
- Put the hazelnuts in the oven and toast them for 12/15 minutes until they turn golden. Let them cool for at least 12 minutes.
- Meanwhile, process the porridge oats to make oat flour.
- Put the hazelnuts to a food processor and process until the mix is totally smooth and creamy. It will take a while and probably you'll have to scrape the nuts from the sides of the food processor at least a couple of times.
- In a bowl, combine the oat flour, the hazelnut butter, maple syrup and add, one at the time, more or less 3 tablespoons of coconut milk (you can take it from the same can you'll later use to make the filling). If you used store-bought hazelnut butter, which is usually more liquid, you might need less coconut milk. If the dough is too dry, you can add more liquid (coconut or almond milk).
- Mix well with your hands and pour the mixture into a greased cake pan (about 22 cm). Press firmly down with your fingers to form a uniform crust,
- Bake for 15/20 minutes in the oven until the crust turns golden.
- Meanwhile prepare the filling. In a bowl, add two tablespoons of tapioca with a little bit of coconut milk. Mix well so that the tapioca dissolves and there are no more lumps.

- In a saucepan, heat the remaining coconut milk and, when it's nice and warm, add chocolate, maple syrup and vanilla powder. Stir constantly with a whisk.
- Continue until the chocolate has melted, then add the coconut milk with the tapioca. Continue stirring for a few minutes over low heat until it thickens. At this point remove from the heat.
- The crust should be ready, so you can leave the oven and let it cool for a few minutes. Pour the coconut filling into the crust.
- Let it cool. Once cold put it in the refrigerator for at least 4 hours.

Pumpkin And Chocolate Cake

Ingredients (10-12 serves)
- 300 gr pumpkin, steamed and puréed
- 130 gr allowed flour / flour mix*
- 4 eggs
- 100 gr maple syrup
- 2 teaspoons baking powder
- 4 teaspoons cocoa powder
- 130 gr dark chocolate (cocoa min. 70%)
- 75 gr extra-virgin coconut oil
- A bit of salt and a bit of vanilla powder

Instructions
- Break the eggs and separate the egg whites from the yolks

- Beat the egg whites until stiff, then put them in the refrigerator.
- Melt the chocolate pieces together with the coconut oil in hot water. Let it cool for 5 minutes.
- In a medium-sized bowl, combine and mix flour, cocoa, vanilla powder, yeast and salt.
- With another bowl, mix well steamed pumpkin, egg yolks and rice syrup using an electric mixer.
- To this mixture, first add the melted chocolate with coconut oil, then the dry ingredients and finally the egg whites, stirring slowly from the bottom to the top.
- Pour all the mixture into a 22 cm diameter baking pan with parchment paper.
- Bake for 40/45 minutes at 180/190°C.

Notes

* You can make your own low FODMAP flour mix using, for instance, 50 gr rice flour, 25 gr cornstarch, 25 gr potato starch, 30 gr oatmeal. Or 65 gr rice flour and 65 gr buckwheat. Depending on the consistency you want to get.

Chocolate Truffles

Ingredients for 25 mini-truffles

- 150 grams dark chocolate (min 70%)
- 100 ml full-fat coconut milk
- 25 grams extra-virgin coconut oil
- 60 grams maple syrup

- A pinch of vanilla powder
- Almond flakes, shredded coconut, hazelnuts and cocoa powder for coating.

Instructions

- Heat the coconut milk in a saucepan and add maple syrup and vanilla.
- When the milk is almost boiling, add the chocolate (previously chopped) and stir until melted. Finally add the coconut oil.
- Place in refrigerator for 3 hours.
- When you have completed the dough, form balls and cover them with coconut, almonds and cocoa.
- In some of them you can place a whole hazelnut and cover with cocoa.

Walnuts And Banana Brownie

Ingredients (8/10 portions)

- 50 grams rice flour
- 30 grams almond meal
- 2 teaspoons of baking powder
- 150 grams extra-virgin coconut oil
- 130 grams Demerara sugar
- 130 grams dark chocolate, chopped (min 70%)
- 4 teaspoons of cocoa powder
- 1 banana, mashed
- 2 large eggs

- 40 grams wanluts (or Brazil nuts), chopped

Instructions

- Melt the extra-virgin coconut oil with the chocolate and let it cool.
- In a bowl mix flour, almond meal, baking powder and cocoa.
- In another bowl beat eggs, sugar and mashed banana with an electric mixer.
- Add the chocolate and coconut oil mixture and mix.
- Add the dry ingredients (flour, almond meal, baking powder and cocoa) and mix well.
- Finally add chopped walnuts.
- Put your mixture in a baking dish (22 cm diameter) and cook for 40/45 minutes at 180/190° C.

Buckwheat And Banana Cake

Ingredients

- 50 grams rice flour
- 50 grams buckwheat flour
- 2 teaspoons baking powder
- 1 tablespoon hazelnut
- 1 tablespoon almonds
- 1 tablespoon sunflower seeds
- 100 grams extra-virgin coconut oil, melted
- 1 egg
- 1 large banana, mashed

- 2 tablespoons maple syrup (or rice syrup)
- 2 tablespoons of coconut yogurt (or lactose-free yogurt)
- Almond flakes, desiccated grated coconut or cacao nibs to garnish

Instructions

- Finely chop the nuts and seeds using a food processor.
- Using an electric mixer, whisk the egg together with coconut oil and mashed banana.
- Add the ground nuts and seeds and maple syrup. Continue whisking with an electric mixer.
- Finally, add the flour, mixed with the baking powder, and the (coconut) yogurt. Stir very well.
- Pour the mixture into a baking dish (18/20 cm diameter) covered with parchment paper.
- Top with almond flakes, grated coconut or cocoa nibs.
- Bake for 35 minutes at 170°C.

Strawberry Clafoutis

Ingredients

- 150-200 gr strawberries
- 60 gr rice flour
- 20 gr potato starch (or mais stach or tapioca)
- 20 gr ground almonds
- 50 ml maple syrup
- 3 eggs

- 200 ml full-fat coconut milk
- Vanilla powder
- Coconut oil or ghee to grease

Instructions

- Wash and cut the strawberries into half.
- Grease a baking dish (22 cm) with coconut oil or ghee and place the strawberries.
- Mix rice flour with potato starch, ground almonds and vanilla powder.
- Using a hand whisk, whisk the eggs with maple syrup.
- Put in coconut milk first and then the dry ingredients. Mix well.
- Pour the mixture over the strawberries and put immediately in the oven.
- Turn on the oven. Insert the pan as soon as it reaches 180 ° C. Then cook for 50/60 minutes.

the # **Part 2**

The Low FODMAP Diet

Do you suffer from symptoms of irritable bowel syndrome IBS or struggle with ongoing digestive problems? Are you concerned about following a bland restrictive diet with limited foods? If so then this recipe and information resource is designed with you in mind.

Each recipe is developed specifically for those following a low-FODMAP diet. They are also designed with families in mind and are quick and easy to prepare and cook.

FODMAP is an acronym for fermentable oligosaccharides, disaccharides, mono-saccharides, and polyols. This style of diet has become the most recommended dietary intervention for irritable bowel syndrome and SIBO (small intestinal bacterial overgrowth). I have been running low FODMAP cookery days in the UK for both practitioners and clients. Many of the most popular recipes from these courses you will find in this book. All the recipes in this book are gluten free and therefore suitable for coeliacs too.

Irritable Bowel Syndrome (IBS)

Irritable bowel syndrome (IBS) is a very common gastrointestinal disorder. It is thought to affect about 11-15% of the global population and can have a long-term effect on your quality of life. In the UK, 1 in 5 people are affected by IBS at some stage in their life. Many people find symptoms impact on their daily activities including work, social events, eating certain foods, and travelling and struggle to lead a 'normal' life.

The symptoms of IBS may include:

- Chronic abdominal pain
- Bloating or swelling of the abdomen
- Diarrhoea, Constipation or erratic bowel habits
- Urgency and incontinence if a toilet is not nearby
- Sensation of incomplete bowel movement

It is often termed a functional disorder because it is not normally associated with any obvious abnormality or tissue damage. However, as it is often associated with other gut disorders, it is important to confirm diagnosis and rule out other conditions via your GP or health care practitioner.

Anyone with symptoms of IBS should be examined for these disorders before going on a low-FODMAP or gluten-free diet with your doctor. However, bear in mind that is possible to have both IBS and another digestive disorder.

Adopting a low FODMAP diet has been shown to improve symptoms in many people with IBS. It may also be helpful for other gut conditions too such as coeliac disease, Crohn's and Colitis. It is recommended that you consult with your health care consultant and registered nutritionist or dietician before embarking on a low-FODMAP diet.

What is a LOW FODMAP Diet?

FODMAPS stands for Fermentable Oligo-saccharides, Di-saccharides, Mono-saccharides and Polyols. These are sugars that are poorly absorbed in the small intestine and fermented by bacteria to produce gas.

FODMAPS are poorly absorbed in the small intestine. These molecules are not absorbed in the small intestine and pass through to the colon – often it is because they cannot be broken down effectively or they are slow to be absorbed. People differ in their abilities to digest and absorb some FODMAPs. Fructose generally is slowly absorbed by everyone but may be slower in certain people. Some people do not make enough of the enzyme lactase to break down lactose while fructans and galacto-oligosaccharides are poorly absorbed in everyone

FODMAPs are also small molecules and often consumed in a concentrated dose. The body attempts to dilute them by forcing water into the gut. This extra fluid can cause diarrhoea and affect the muscular movements of the gut.

FODMAPS are also food for the bacteria that live in our gut. The bacteria in the small intestine and colon feed on these molecules and quickly break them down which produces hydrogen, carbon dioxide and methane – i.e. these short chains are fermented quickly.

Most meals will contain a range of these fermentable carbohydrates – their effect is cumulative and this can lead to symptoms such as bowel distension, loose stools etc. For more details on FODMAPs please see the research by The Monash University, Dept of Gastroenterology, Monash University, Australia. www.med.monash.edu

Types of FODMAPs

People may react to one group of FODMAPS or all of them.

Oligosaccharides

These include fructans and the glacto-oligosaccharides (GOS)

Fructans are chains of fructose molecules with a glucose molecule at the end. The main dietary sources include wheat products (breads, cereals and pasta) some vegetables such as onions. Additional sources of fructans are the fructo-oligosaccharides (FOS) and inulins that are added to foods such as certain yogurts and milks. No one can digest fructans so if you have IBS it is recommended to limit you intake. They are considered a problem if they contain more then 0.2grams of fructans per serving of food for cereals and 0.3g fructans per serving of other foods.

Galacto Oligosaccharides (GOS) are short chain molecules formed from galactose sugars joined together with a fructose and glucose at the end. Raffinose and stachyose are the most common GOS in foods – they are particularly evident in beans, legumes, lentils etc

High GOS foods are those that contain more than 0.2 grams per serving. Some people may be able to cope with a small amount of canned and rinsed chickpeas for example

High GOS foods includes all beans and pulses including lentils and soybean (except soy sauce GF and tofu, soy yogurt)

Disaccharides

The main one is lactose. Lactose is a double sugar that occurs naturally in animal milks including cows, sheep, and goats. Made up of two sugars glucose and galactose it is broken down in the small intestine into its component sugars by an enzyme called lactase.

Lactose intolerant people have low levels of lactase and can only break down a small amount. However it is likely they still produce some so may not need to exclude it completely from their diet.

A lactose free diet is NOT the same as a dairy free diet. Lactose is present in varying amounts in milk and milk products such as kefir, yogurt, ice cream, cream, cheese. Cream contains a minimal amount of lactose and hard and ripened cheeses (cheddar, parmesan, camembert, edam, gouda, blue and mozzarella) and butter are virtually lactose free. Most people with a lactose malabsorption can handle up to 4g of lactose per serving without experiencing problems. A thin spread of butter and a small amount of cream or milk in coffee may therefore be tolerated.

High lactose foods are those with 4g or more per serving. Moderate contain 1-4 grams per serving and low lactose foods are those with less than 1g per serving

FOOD	LACTOSE (grams)
Whole milk 1 cup	16
Low fat milk 1 cup	15
Skimmed milk 1 cup	13
Evaporated milk ½ cup	13

Cottage cheese ½ cup	8
Low fat yogurt 6 oz	6
Whole milk yogurt 6oz	6
Cheesecake 1 small slice	6
Milk chocolate 2 oz	6
Ice cream 2 scoops	4
White sauce 2tbsp	2
Full fat cream cheese 1tbsp	1
Sour cream 1tbsp	0.5
Cream 1tbsp	0.4
Butter 1tbsp	0.1
Hard Cheese 1oz	0.1

Choosing Low Lactose and / or dairy free alternatives.

Hard and ripened cheeses e.g blue, brie, cheddar, edam, Emmental, feta, gorgonzola, gouda, Monterey Jack, Mozzarella, Parmesan, Pecorino, Stilton, Swiss Cheese, soy cheese (up to 2 oz)

Nut yogurt, coconut yogurt, soy yogurt (without inulin if FOS a problem) Alpro soy milk plain does not contain inulin. Co-Yo plain coconut yogurt is also free of sweeteners or thickeners.

For ice cream and milk options choose soy (check labels) or almond or coconut ice cream, lactose free options. Other options Lactose free milk, soy milk, rice, oat, almond, quinoa milks (check sugars added)

Monosaccharides

Mono means one, and saccharide means sugar. So these are simple sugars. The most important is the role of excess fructose.

Fructose is a single sugar often referred to as fruit sugar – found in fruits, honey, high fructose corn syrup, a component of table sugar (also called sucrose) and found in some vegetables (sugar snap peas) and wheat.

When fructose occurs with glucose it is well absorbed because the glucose aids it across the bowel. If fructose is in higher concentrations then absorption is slower. When it is incomplete it is known as fructose malabsorption. Foods are often considered a problem if they contain more than 0.2g fructose in excess of glucose per serving.

So it is not just about the amount of fructose a food contains but the ratio of fructose and glucose. It is only generally a problem when fructose is MUCH Higher then glucose.

It is also a good idea to space out fruit consumption so only eat a little in one sitting.

Example

Honey contains 40g fructose per 100g, and 30 grams of glucose per 100g – this means and excess of 10 grams per serving = **problem**

Mango contains 2 grams fructose per 100g and 1.5 grams glucose per 100g = 0.5 excess = **problem**

Kiwi contains 4 grams fructose per 100g and 4g glucose = no excess = not a problem

POLYOLS

These are sugar alcohols – often added to foods, chewing gum, excess can have a laxative effect. Foods with more than 0.5g per serving are often a problem. Look out for sorbitol, mannitol, xylitol, polydextrose, isomalt, ethyritol

Testing For Malabsorption

Though all FODMAPs may trigger symptoms of IBS, there are breath hydrogen tests available to determine individual sensitivity to certain sugars, especially fructose, lactose, and sorbitol. Breath tests are not a prerequisite for following the low-FODMAP diet but can be helpful in planning it. Your GP or health care practitioner should be able to arrange these tests. The test measures the amount of gas in the breath after swallowing a measured amount of sugar to produce gases including hydrogen and methane. These gases are absorbed across the intestine carried through the bloodstream to the lungs and exhaled.

Detection of a rise in breath hydrogen confirms the test sugar (fructose, lactose or sorbitol) has been malabsorbed and would indicate which elements would need to be restricted in the diet. Only these sugars can be formally tested.

Following A Low FODMAP Diet.

Remember that FODMAP diet is not a diet to follow for life. It is intended to isolate offending foods and reduce symptoms while you focus on gut support and / or anti-microbial support.

Normally it is recommended you follow a strict low FODMAP diet for 4-8 weeks or until you are symptom free. After this time the re-introduction phase is recommended (see below).

Low FODMAP Foods

The following table outlines the foods to include and those to avoid. This is based on the work by Monash University. Please see our shopping list for a summary of key foods to include in your diet.

FOOD GROUP	HIGH FODMAPS - AVOID	LOW FODMAP - INCLUDE
FLOURS AND GRAINS	Barley, bulgar, chickpea flour, couscous, durum, kamut, multigrain flour, wheat flour, soy flour, semolina, wheat bran, wheat germ, rye, triticale, kamut, pea flour (in small amounts may be tolerable)	Arrrowroot, buckwheat, corn, gluten free flour mixes, millet, oat bran, polenta, sorghum, tapioca, sago, rice, rice bran, potato flour, quinoa, wild rice, popcorn, ground rice
CEREALS	Wheat based and mixed grain cereals and muesli	Rice cereal, buckwheat porridge, corn based cereals, gluten free cereals
PASTA AND NOODLES	Wheat, barley and rye containing noodles and pasta, gnocchi	Mung bean noodles, rice noodles, buckwheat, gluten free pasta
BREADS, COOKIES ETC	Breads, including sourdough, breadcrumbs, pastries,	Gluten free breads, corn tortillas, plain rice cakes, rice

	cakes, cookies, croissants, muffins etc containing wheat, rye and barley	crackers, gluten free crackers, corn taco shells
DAIRY	Regular milk, ice cream, soft cheeses, yogurt	Lactose free milk, lactose free ice cream, soy milk, rice, quinoa and oat milks, nut milks, butter, hard and ripened cheeses, gelato and sorbets made from suitable fruits
MEAT AND VEGETARIAN OPTIONS PROTEIN	Certain sausages check for onion powder or dehydrated vegetable powders	Bacon, eggs, fish, meat, poultry, tempeh, tofu
NUTS NAD SEEDS	Pistachios and cashew	All others (no more than handful of 2tbsp nut butter with each serving)
VEGETABLES	Artichokes globe and Jerusalem, asparagus, cauliflower, garlic, leek, onions, spring onion (white parts), snow peas, sugar snap peas, shallots	Alfalfa sprouts, bamboo shoots, bean sprouts, pepper, bok choy, broccoli, carrot, Chinese cabbage, lettuce, green beans parsnip, Swiss chard, squash except butternut,

		turnips, watercress, courgette, yams, potato, pumpkin, cucumber, aubergine, green part of spring onion
FRUITS	Apples, apricot, Asian pear, pear, blackberries, cherries, figs, persimmon, watermelon, white peaches, prunes, tamarillo, plums, peaches, mango nectarines	Banana, blueberries, cantaloupe melon, durian, cranberries, citrus fruits, passion fruit, papaya, pineapple, tomatoes, strawberries, raspberries, honeydew melon
SPREADS AND CONDIMENTS	Most commercial relishes, chutneys, gravies, stock, sauces, dressings, bouillon cubes	Jam and marmalade, mayonnaise, mustard, soy sauce, garlic free sauces, vinegar
Sweeteners	Agave, honey, high fructose corn syrup, fruit juice concentrate, xylitol, mannitol, sorbitol, maltitol	Sucrose – table sugar, icing sugar, maple syrup, molasses, rice syrup, brown sugar, stevia
DRINKS	Apple, pear and mango juices, other fruit juices if more than ½ cup, chicory based coffee,	Water, mineral, soda water, sugar sweetened drinks, most teas, coffee,

		dandelion tea and coffee, rum, watch out for mixers in alcohol drinks, beer may also be problem, sweet wines, sparkling, dessert wines	most alcohol
FATS		Do not use apple sauce as a replacer	Butter, ghee, lard, margarines, garlic infused oil
OTHER		NOT Onion powder or garlic powders	Baking powder, bicarbonate of soda, cocoa, coconut gelatine, salt, xanthum gum, fresh and dried herbs, chives, ginger

The Reintroduction Phase

There is an order to the reintroduction phase – start with small amounts then gradually build up to avoid adverse effects

The first group to test is the Polyol. To do this most people choose to try an avocado or apricots (these contain sorbitol). A recommended amount is ½ avocado or 2 fresh apricots – if you experience any symptoms stop and wait until you are symptom free before trying again or trying a new food.

After the avocado / apricot try some mushroom, and if this is tolerated try cauliflower – see the table below. It is recommended you do this with the help of a qualified nutritionist or dietician.

Once you have tested this group move onto the next group – use the following order below:

FODMAP GROUP	FOOD TO INTRODUCE
Polyols	¼ ripe avocado (contains sorbitol) 2 medium fresh apricots or 4 dried apricot halves (contains sorbitol) ½ cup mushrooms (contains manitol) ½ cup Cauliflower (contains manitol)
LACTOSE	½ to 1 cup of milk or 6oz yogurt
FRUTCOSE	½ mango or 1tsp honey
FRUCTANS	1 slice white bread then move up to 2 slices white bread or 1 garlic clove then build up to testing ¼ onion this is tested last as they have a high

	fructan content
GALACTO OLIGOSACCHARIDES	½ cup lentil, kidney beans, baked beans or chickpeas

Key points when re-introducing foods

- Test only one FODMAP group at a time
- Choose an amount of food that reflects a portion size – too little or too much may affect results
- Where possible choose a food that contains mainly one type of FODMAP
- Continue to restrict all other FODMAPs until your tolerance or intolerance is confirmed
- Maintain a normal intake of alcohol and caffeine if you consume these – do not increase foods that you think may also be a problem for you
- Challenge with one FODMAP group per week
- Eat the challenge food at least twice during the test week unless reaction in the first attempt in which case stop

If you don't get symptoms

Increase the range of foods that contain the FODMAP you are testing and assess response

Or

maintain the same amount and type of food you have tested and then move on to the next FODMAP group challenge

If you get symptoms

Remove the suspect food and wait until the symptoms are free again then reduce the serving size by half and try again

Or try another food from within the same FODMAP group to confirm it is a problem

Or assume that this type of FODMAP is a problem for you and restrict these

The dose of FODMAP is vital – if symptoms occur then try half the amount and repeat but wait until you are symptom free before doing this. Consider a challenge again in the future as sensitivity may change over time.

SHOPPING GUIDE – LOW FODMAP FOODS

For further details of FODMAPs please see the research by The Monash University, Dept of Gastroenterology, Monash University, Australia. www.med.monash.edu

It is also important to remember it is often the quantity of foods eaten that causes a problem. Therefore portion size is important and how much of certain types of sugars you eat over the day.

It is important to check labels carefully – many processed foods will contain certain flavourings that can aggravate symptoms – watch out for the following: onion, garlic, onion salt, garlic salt, commercial stocks and stock cubes, stock powder

What About Sugars?

The following are safe on FODMAP diet – however for health keep to a minimum

- Caster sugar / table sugar / brown sugar / jaggery
- Stevia
- Maple syrup
- **Golden syrup**

Avoid xylitol, agave nectar, coconut sugar, honey, high fructose corn syrup. Watch out for products that contain concentrated fruit juices or dried fruits. If fructose is listed as one of the first foods in the ingredients list then it is likely to be high in fructose so avoid.

The following foods are safe on a low FODMAP diet

VEGETABLES	FRUITS
Aubergine	Banana
< ¼ cup artichoke hearts canned in water or vinegar	Blueberry
	Cantaloupe melon
alfalfa	Durian
Bamboo shoots	Dragon fruit
Beans, green	Grapefruit < ½ medium
Bean sprouts	Grapes
Beetroot – limit to 2 slices	Honeydew melon
Broccoli – limit to < ½ cup	Kiwifruit
Cabbage, savoy < ½ cup	Lemon
Carrot	Lime
Courgette	Lychee < 5
Celery – limit to ½ stalk	Papaya
Cucumber	Orange,
Fennel bulb < ½ cup	Satsuma
Ginger	Passionfruit
Lettuce	Pineapple
Olives	Pomegranate – ½ small
Okra	Raspberry
Parsnip	Rhubarb
Peas, green – limit to <1/4 cup	Strawberry
Potato	
Rocket	
Spinach	
Spring onion – green part only	
Seaweed nori sheets	
Swede	

Spring greens Turnip Tomato – all types Sweet potato Butternut squash < ¼ cup Pumpkin Red peppers Water chestnuts	
MILK PRODUCTS Hard cheese – including feta, brie Haloumi cheese < 100g Lactose free milk Rice milk Soy milk – check labels Lactose free yogurt Soy yogurt – check labels Coconut yogurt Almond milk – check labels Hemp milk – check labels Coconut milk – check labels	**PROTEIN FOODS** Poultry Red meat Fish Seafood Tofu
CEREALS AND GRAINS – KEEP LOW OR AVOID COMPLETELY **IF ON PALEO STYLE OF EATING** Gluten free breads (check dairy free) Cornflakes	**Nuts and seeds** – limit portion to 1 small handful, about 10 nuts Avoid cashew and pistachio Almonds Pecans Hazelnuts Flaxseed Chia

Cornflour Gluten free flour Gluten free muesli Oats and oat bran Gluten free pasta Rice Quinoa Amaranth Polenta Corn crackers Rice cakes	Sunflower Pumpkin Pine nuts Peanuts Sesame seeds Walnuts
BEVERAGES Alcohol is an irritant to the gut – limit alcohol. FODMAPs are found in some wines and cider. Rum is high in fructose. Watch out for juice blends and topical juices, high fructose corn syrup, honey sweetened drinks Be mindful of gluten containing drinks Limit fruit juice to ½ glass – the safest are orange juice and cranberry No chicory, Caro, Carob, barley cup, dandelion coffee drinks A little red wine can be used esp. in cooking e.g stews	**FLAVOURINGS** Fresh herbs The green tops of spring onions Chives Chilli Garlic infused oil – simply peel and cut garlic and add to olive oil to seep the flavour. Discard the garlic Ginger Lemon and lime juice and zest Maple syrup Salt and pepper Spices – cumin, coriander etc. Avoid seasoning mixes Make up your own stock by simmering bones with carrot, celery, garlic infused oil, salt and pepper Vinegars – keep to 1-2tbsp only per portion

	Fish sauce
	Tamari soy sauce
	Mustard
	Peanut butter
	Tahini
	Sesame oil

Tweaking the Diet to Suit Dietary Requirements
Vegetarian & Vegan Diets

If you are following a low FODMAP diet and also avoid meat or animal products it is important to ensure your diet contains sufficient protein. This can be challenging because beans and pulses which can form an important part of a vegetarian / vegan diet are also high in GOS and fructans.

Vegetarian sources of protein include: eggs, tofu (plain, unflavoured), soy milk (check labels), tempeh (plain, unflavoured), eggs, quinoa, lactose free yogurt, lactose free milk, hard cheese (small quantities), some nuts and seeds (including tahini paste). Vegans will need to pay particular attention as they will also be excluding eggs and dairy products. Soy milk made from whole soy beans is often higher in FODMAPs than those made from soy protein so do check labels carefully. Pure protein isolate is also suitable on a low FODMAP diet – whey isolate, pea protein isolate, hemp and egg proteins may therefore be useful additions to the diet but check labels as many brands will contain sugars and sweeteners and inulin making them unsuitable.

Paleo Diet

The paleo diet is based upon how we ate before our modern day diet of processed foods, sugars, salts, high fructose corn syrups and modified produce. A strict Paleo approach removes all grains, dairy and legumes (beans and pulses) from the diet. Some will also reduce or eliminate their intake of nightshade vegetables like peppers, tomatoes, and aubergine initially particularly if they suffer with an autoimmune condition. Protein rich foods (meats, fish, eggs) are all suitable on a FODMAP diet. However certain vegetables will need to be avoided (see tables above) and those following a paleo diet may need to watch the quantity of nuts and seeds consumed which can be high in some paleo recipes. Some people find they struggle with obtaining sufficient fibre in their diet as they avoid all grains, beans, and pulses. Good paleo fibre rich sources include potato, sweet potato (1/2 cup), carrots, leafy green vegetables, swede, ground flaxseed, ground chia seed, shelled hemp seeds.

Example Meal Options

The following are examples of meals suitable for a low FODMAP diet. If you have specific requirements (e.g paleo, vegan, vegetarian) look at our recipes, which are labelled appropriately for you. All the recipes are gluten free and suitable for those with Coeliac Disease.

Breakfast Options

Eggs With Low FODMAP Vegetables And Sweet Potato Rosti

Omelette With Vegetables – Low FODMAP e.g Spinach, Green Beans, Tomatoes

Poached eggs with spinach

Granola – See Recipe

Muffins – See Recipe

Frittata – using sweet potato and low FODMAP vegetables

Olives, Smoked Salmon and Vegetables

Quinoa Porridge Made With Almond Milk

Millet Porridge With Fresh Berries

Green Smoothie – blend up banana, coconut milk, spinach leaves, lemon and ginger

Green Juice – lemon, parsley, spinach or kale, celery, cucumber, pineapple (small piece only)

Gluten free Oats* or Quinoa Flakes with almond milk or low lactose milk (if tolerated) plus 1tbsp mixed seeds

Plain soy yogurt (low inulin), homemade coconut yogurt (to avoid xylitol) berries plus 1tbsp mixed seeds

Scrambled tofu with gluten free toast or paleo bread

Gluten free sausages, tomatoes, wilted spinach

Pancetta baked eggs

GF pancakes with berries and soy or coconut yogurt

Paleo porridge – eggs, coconut flour, coconut milk

Amaranth porridge

Useful Snacks

1tbsp nuts or seeds

Plain soy yogurt or coconut yogurt

Rice cake with nut butter, slices of beef

30g hard cheese and raw cracker

Homemade kale crisps

Handful of olives

Carrot sticks and 1tbsp natural peanut butter

Sushi

Lunch / Dinner Options (see recipes for ideas)

Quinoa salad with protein e.g fish, chicken

Omelette with low FODMAP vegetables or salad

Homemade soup using FODMAP friendly vegetables

Poached fish or chicken with vegetables and sweet potato wedges

Small baked potato with tuna and homemade mayonnaise and salad

Roast meats with vegetables and potato

Frittata with salad

Sushi

Rice paper rolls

Vietnamese Beef Salad

* note not all coeliacs can tolerate certified gluten free oats. If these are a problem for you switch to a paleo style recipe or use quinoa, rice or buckwheat flakes instead

RECIPES

Drinks

Anti-inflammatory turmeric shake

Cinnamon Hot Chocolate

Breads and Breakfasts

Almond Butter & Banana Muffins

Quinoa Protein Porridge

Butternut Squash / Pumpkin and Cinnamon Granola

Bacon, Sundried and Courgette Frittata

Eggs Muffin Cups Wrapped In Prosciutto

Breakfast Burritos

Sundried Tomato and Olive Muffins

Paleo Focaccia Bread

Chocolate Banana Paleo Bread

Herb Blinis With Hot Smoked Salmon And Aioli

Soups

Creamy Carrot Ginger Soup

Roasted Red Pepper And Tomato Soup

Snacks and Condiments

Digestive Mix

Coconut Oil Mayonnaise

Tomato Ketchup

Easy Rosemary Flaxseed Crackers

Parmesan Crackers

Cheese Rice Crackers

Chocolate Hazelnut Spread

Curry Flavoured Nuts

Meat Dishes

Paleo Sausage and Sun Dried Tomato Quiche

Warming Gingered Beef Stew

Seared Lamb With A Minted Dressing and Green beans

Poultry

Crispy Almond Paleo Chicken

Sicilian Chicken Quinoa Salad

Sticky Chicken with Cucumber Salad

Turkey & Bacon Meatloaf

Stuffed Roasted Red Peppers

Fish

Bacon Wrapped Salmon with Caponata

Pan Fried Cod with Gremolata

Salads

Lemon Crab & Prawn Salad With Lemon Dressing

Asian Kale Salad

Creamy Caesar Style Salad

Vietnamese Beef Salad

Thai Pork and Pineapple Salad

Carrot & Courgette Spiral Salad with Creamy Red Pepper Sauce

Desserts / Treats

Blueberries With Coconut Cream

Raspberry Hazelnut Tart

Lemon Bars

Chocolate Chip Ice Cream

Almond Kheer

Sweet Potato Brownies

Chocolate Fridge Fudge

RECIPES

Drinks

Anti-Inflammatory Turmeric Shake

A simple alternative to the morning smoothie – you can use lactose free milk, coconut milk or almond milk. Some milk or coconut kefir may also be low in lactose and could be a useful alternative. Freezing the banana creates a wonderful creamy texture to the shake but is optional.

Gluten Free, Suitable for Vegetarians, Paleo

Serves 2

1 large banana, sliced and frozen

2tsp Maple Syrup

300ml almond milk or coconut milk or milk kefir (if tolerated)

1 scoop protein powder (isolate), optional

1tsp ground flaxseed

2tsp chia seeds

2 tsp turmeric powder

Pinch of black pepper

Drizzle of omega blended oil

1/2 tsp cinnamon powder

1. Simply blend all the ingredients together and serve immediately.

Cinnamon Hot Chocolate

A wonderful warming recipe

Gluten Free, Dairy Free, Suitable for Vegetarians, Suitable for Vegans, Paleo

Serves 2

3 Tbsp Cocoa powder

1tbsp Maple Syrup

1 tsp. cinnamon

1 pinch cayenne (or more if you like it spicy!)

2 cups of milk, e.g almond milk or coconut milk.

1. Mix the cocoa powder and cinnamon together in a small bowl with the maple syrup to form a smooth paste.
2. Spoon a little of the milk into the paste to slacken slightly. Warm up the remaining milk in a small sauce pan, keeping the heat on low.
3. Gradually stir in the chocolate paste mix and whisk until completely dissolved.

Breads And Breakfast Options

Almond Butter & Banana Muffins

A simple muffin sweetened with fruit only. These are great for snacks and packed lunches or for a grab and go breakfast. You could add some protein powder to this if wished e.g soy isolate, hemp protein powder or whey protein powder if tolerated

Gluten Free, Dairy Free, Suitable for Vegetarians, Paleo

Makes 8

4 bananas

4 eggs

1/2 cup / 125g almond butter

2 tbsp coconut oil, melted

1 tsp vanilla

1/2 cup / 55g coconut flour

2 tsp cinnamon

1/2 tsp nutmeg

1 tsp baking powder

1 tsp bicarbonate of soda

Pinch of sea salt

1. Preheat the oven to 180C, gas mark 4. Line a muffin tin with cases. In a blender or food processor combine bananas, eggs, almond butter, coconut oil, and vanilla.
2. Add in the coconut flour, cinnamon, nutmeg, baking powder, soda, and salt. Blend into the wet mixture, scraping down the sides with a spatula.
3. Spoon into the muffin cases.
4. Bake for 20-25 minutes, until a toothpick comes out clean.
5. Best stored in the fridge or frozen

VARIATIONS – cocoa powder is FODMAP friendly – use 1tbsp. You could also stir in 2tbsp chopped walnuts to the mixture if wished.

Quinoa Protein Porridge

This could be made with millet grain too. A warming alternative to porridge.

Gluten Free, Dairy Free, Suitable for Vegetarians

Serves 2

1 cup dairy free milk – almond or coconut (check labels)

1 cup water

1/2 cup quinoa

1 banana, sliced

½ teaspoon ground cinnamon

1 teaspoon vanilla extract

1 tablespoon ground flaxseed

1 scoop pure protein powder isolate - optional

1. Rinse the quinoa under cold running water.
2. Place the quinoa and water in a pan and bring to the boil.
3. Reduce the heat then cover and cook for 10 minutes until just soft.
4. Add the milk, banana, cinnamon, flaxseeds, protein if using and vanilla.
5. Cook for 5 minutes until creamy. Add a little more milk if needed for a creamier texture.
6. Spoon into serving bowls.

Butternut Squash / Pumpkin And Cinnamon Granola

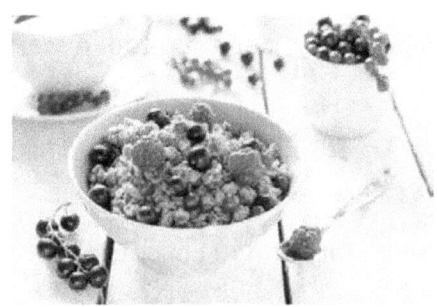

Note that most nuts are medium FODMAPs so watch portion sizes – if you are following the exclusion diet I suggest just one handful of this recipe in one sitting only. You can use this granola as a topping for soy yogurt or low lactose yogurt too. Alternatively you could add some gluten free oats, quinoa or buckwheat flakes to replace some of the nuts in this mixture. Make up a batch and store in an airtight container for 1 week or keep in the fridge for longer.

Gluten Free, Dairy Free, Suitable for Vegetarians, Suitable for Vegans, Paleo*

Serves 8

1 cup / 125g quinoa flakes, buckwheat flakes or gluten free oats (*for paleo option use 1 cup ground almonds)

180g / 1½ cup sliced / flaked almonds

70g / 1 cup unsweetened coconut flakes

125g / 1 cup pumpkin seeds or mixture of seeds e.g sunflower, sesame and pumpkin

2tbsp flaxseed ground

125g / 1 cup walnuts, chopped

½ cup / 60g coconut oil melted

2 Tbsp maple syrup

1tbsp vanilla extract

Pinch of sea salt

115g / ½ cup pumpkin or butternut squash pureed from a can or you can bake in the oven then puree

2 tsp ground cinnamon

Serve with mixed berries and coconut yogurt or soy yogurt

1. Preheat the oven to 180C, gas mark 4 and line a baking sheet with parchment paper.
2. In a large bowl combine flakes (or ground almond), coconut flakes, almonds, pumpkin seeds and pecans.
3. In a blender, combine the pumpkin, coconut oil, maple syrup and cinnamon.
4. Add the wet ingredients to the dry ingredients and stir until dry ingredients are thoroughly coated.
5. Spread the granola in a thin layer on the baking sheet.
6. Cook for 30 minutes stirring occasionally to prevent burning.

Bacon, Sundried Tomato And Courgette Frittata

A wonderful option served hot or cold. If you pour the mixture into a traybake tin you can cut it into squares and take a portion with you to work for lunch as well.

Gluten Free, Paleo* (*omit cheese)

Serves 4

8 slices of streaky bacon, cut into dice

2 medium courgettes, grated

6 sundried tomatoes, chopped

100g grated hard cheese, lactose free cheese or soy cheese

6 large eggs, lightly beaten

6 cherry tomatoes, halved

Pinch of cayenne pepper

Salt and freshly ground black pepper

1. Preheat the oven to 180C, gas mark 4. Grease an 20cm / 8inch cake tin or small traybake and line with greaseproof baking parchment.
2. Cook the bacon in a frying pan until crispy. Remove from the heat and drain.
3. Combine the bacon, courgette, sundried tomatoes, cheese and eggs in a large bowl. Season with salt and pepper and cayenne. Pour into the baking dish, top with the cherry tomatoes and bake for 20 to 25 minutes, until firm and golden brown.
4. Remove from the oven and let stand for 5 minutes before slicing.

Eggs Muffin Cups Wrapped In Prosciutto

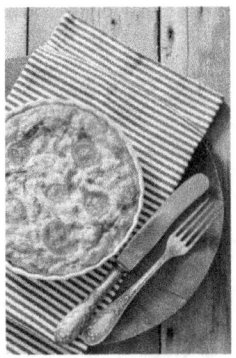

Easy to assemble and portable too – serve hot or cold

Gluten Free, Dairy Free, Paleo

Serves 4

4 eggs

4 slices of bacon

salt and pepper

1 tomato, chopped

chopped chives

1. Preheat the oven to 180C, gas mark 4
2. Lightly grease a muffin pan and begin by taking one slice of uncooked bacon at a time, wrap the inside of a muffin cup to create a ring. Repeat with the remaining slices of bacon.
3. Sprinkle the tomatoes and chives into the muffin cups, and crack an egg into each muffin case. Season with salt and pepper.

4. Bake in the oven for 15-20 minutes. Or until eggs are cooked to your liking – you may only need 15 minutes for a runny yolk

Breakfast Burritos

A delicious paleo style recipe – you can alter the fillings according to what is available.

Gluten Free, Dairy Free, Paleo

Serves 4

3 eggs

½ cup about 100ml coconut milk (check labels)

2tbsp coconut flour, sifted

1tsp coconut oil

½ tsp arrowroot

pinch of salt

Coconut oil or olive oil for pan

Filling

2tbsp olive oil

350g rump steak, finely chopped

½ red chilli, seeds removed, finely chopped

1 tomato, diced

dash Tabasco sauce

pinch cayenne pepper

small handful fresh coriander, chopped

1. Make the tortillas. Whisk the tortilla ingredients together in a bowl. Let the mixture sit for 10 minutes while the pan

heats so the coconut flour can absorb the liquid, then whisk again.
2. Heat a crepe pan or frying pan over a medium-high heat.
3. Melt a small amount of oil in the pan, swirling to coat the bottom and sides.
4. Pour ¼ of the batter into the hot pan, turning the pan in a circular motion with one hand so to spread the batter thinly around the pan.
5. Cook for 1 minute until the edges start to lift and turn golden. Gently work a spatula under the crepe and flip it over. Cook on the second side for 15 seconds and turn out on a plate.
6. Repeat with the remaining batter
7. To make the filling sauté the steak, chilli and tomato and fry until the meat is golden and cooked through, about 4 minutes. Add the remaining ingredients and season to taste.
8. To assemble the burrito, place the warmed tortillas on serving plates and divide the steak between them. You could top with a little lettuce too. Roll up to serve

Sundried Tomato And Olive Muffins

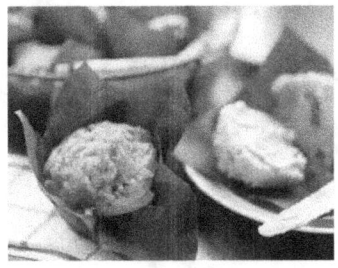

A fabulous healthy snack and perfect for packed lunches. Full of Meditterrean flavours these are rich and satisfying. Delicious warm from the oven or served with bacon and grilled vegetables for a breakfast style brunch

Gluten Free, Dairy Free, Suitable for Vegetarians

Makes 7 muffins

Preparation time: 10 minutes

Cooking time: 30 minutes

225g self raising gluten free flour

1 tsp gluten-free baking powder

¼ tsp xanthan gum

½ tsp salt

80g hard cheese or low lactose cheese, grated

40g or 5 drained, bottled sun-dried tomatoes, finely chopped

8 olives, pitted and chopped

4 fresh basil leaves, finely chopped

75g dairy-free spread or coconut oil, melted

2 large eggs, beaten

1 tbsp sun dried tomato paste

150ml dairy-free milk or lactose free milk (check labels)

1. Preheat the oven to 180°C, gas 4. Line a muffin tin with paper cases

2. Place the flour, baking powder, xanthan gum and salt into a mixing bowl and stir thoroughly. Add the dairy-free cheese, sun-dried tomatoes, olives and basil leaves and mix well.
3. Mix together the melted spread or oil, eggs, tomato purée and dairy-free milk.
4. Pour the egg mixture into the flour mixture and gently mix in. Spoon the mixture into the muffin cases.
5. Bake for about 25-30 minutes until golden brown. Remove from the oven and place on a cool rack. Delicious eaten hot or cold

Paleo Focaccia Bread

Vary the flavourings according to taste. You can add a little garlic olive to it if wished.

Gluten Free, Dairy Free, Suitable for Vegetarians, Paleo

Makes 1 loaf

4 large eggs

1/4 cup coconut cream - taken from the top of a can of coconut milk

1/4 cup coconut flour

1/2 teaspoon bicarbonate of soda

1tsp baking powder

Handful of chopped fresh herbs - thyme, or rosemary work well.

Olive oil, for brushing

Additional coarse sea salt, for topping

Chopped olives and cherry tomatoes for topping

1. Preheat oven to 180C, gas mark 4.
2. Beat the eggs with the coconut cream until smooth. In a medium bowl, combine the coconut flour, salt, baking powder and soda. Add the egg mixture to the flour and stir until well combined. Make sure there are no lumps
3. Stir in a handful of fresh herbs e.g rosemary
4. Line a round cake tin or small square traybake tin with parchment and spread the batter in the pan. Drizzle with olive oil. Top with herbs, olives and cherry tomatoes.
5. Bake for 15-20 minutes until top is lightly browned. Remove from the oven and brush with more olive oil. Cool before slicing and serving.

Chocolate Banana Paleo Bread

Vary the ingredients – you can add grated courgette to this basic recipe.

Gluten Free, Dairy Free, Suitable for Vegetarians, Paleo

1 ¾ cups almonds ground up until fine in a blender or food processor

3tbsp raw cacao powder or 2tbsp cocoa powder

¼ cup coconut flour

1tsp bicarbonate of soda

¼ cup / 60ml olive oil

5 eggs

1 banana

1tbsp maple syrup or pinch of stevia

1. Heat the oven to 180C gas mark 4

2. Place the almond flour, cocoa powder, coconut flour and bicarbonate of soda in a bowl.
3. Mix well. In a blender blend up the olive oil, eggs, banana and maple syrup. Add the wet ingredients to the bowl and beat well
4. Pour the mixture into a loaf tin and bake in the oven for 40 minutes until golden and firm

Herb Blinis With Hot Smoked Salmon And Aioli

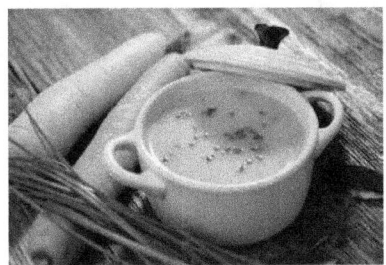

These wonderful gluten free blinis, flavoured with fresh herbs are simple and quick to prepare. Despite its name, buckwheat isn't a grain but a fruit seed related to rhubarb. It contains all eight essential amino acids, making it a good source of protein. Accompany with hot smoked or smoked salmon and a little aioli for a perfect canapé or party dish but equally delicious as indulgent breakfast or brunch.

Gluten Free, Dairy Free

Makes 20 blinis

Storage: Make in advance and keep in the fridge for up to 2 days. Warm through in the oven. Freeze in batches for up to 1 month.

Preparation time: 10 minutes

Cooking time: 15-20 minutes

100g/4oz buckwheat flour

1tsp gluten free baking powder

1/2tsp sea salt

Freshly ground black pepper

1 egg, separated

150ml/5floz milk alternative or lactose free milk

1tsp grated lemon zest

1tbsp chopped dill

1tbsp chopped parsley

1tbsp olive oil or coconut butter

225g / 8oz hot smoked salmon, flaked or smoked salmon

Aioli

2 free-range egg yolks

pinch of mustard powder

Salt and pepper

100ml/ 3 ½ floz light olive oil

100ml / 3 ½ floz omega blended oil or olive oil

Juice of ½ lemon

1. To make the aioli, put the egg yolks in a food processor, add a pinch of mustard powder, salt and pepper and pulse briefly. With the machine running, gradually trickle in the oil to form a thick smooth emulsion. Pulse in the lemon juice. Spoon into a bowl and chill until needed.
2. For the blinis place the flour, baking powder, seasoning, egg yolk, milk alternative and lemon zest in a bowl. Using a hand-held blender process to form a smooth batter.
3. Whisk the egg white until stiff then fold into the batter with the herbs.
4. Heat the oil in a frying pan. Place spoonfuls of the mixture into the pan. Cook for 2-3 minutes on each side. Repeat with the rest of the mixture.
5. To serve top each blinis with a little smoked salmon and a spoonful of aioli

Soups

Creamy Carrot Ginger Soup

The addition of silken tofu provides a wonderful creamy texture to this soup. For a paleo option try blending in some coconut cream at the end. If you have a vitamix you can make this in the blender. Otherwise cook in a pan before blending.

Gluten Free, Dairy Free, Suitable for Vegetarians, Suitable for Vegans, Paleo

Serves 2

2 tablespoons olive or coconut oil

4 medium carrots, peeled, chopped

1 celery stalk, chopped

1/2 teaspoon sea salt

pinch white pepper

1 tablespoon fresh ginger root

125g silken tofu or use ¼ cup coconut cream (check labels)

450ml vegetable or chicken broth (check labels if not homemade)

Chopped chives to garnish

1. Heat the oil in a pan and add the carrots and celery. Sauté for 5 minutes to soften.
2. Add the remaining ingredients and cook until the carrot is soft.
3. Blend until smooth and creamy.
4. Sprinkle over the chives to serve.

Roasted Red Pepper And Tomato Soup

A simple store cupboard soup recipe. You can either roast the peppers yourself or use those in a jar (check labels)

Gluten Free, Dairy Free, Suitable for Vegetarians, Suitable for Vegans, Paleo (use coconut cream)

Serves 4

3 red peppers, halved and deseeded

1 tbsp olive oil or coconut oil

1 red chilli, chopped and deseeded

400g (14oz) can chopped tomatoes

1 tbsp sundried tomato paste

425ml (¾ pint) fresh vegetable stock, preferably homemade or chicken stock

275g (10oz) silken tofu or use ¼ cup of coconut cream

1tbsp fresh herbs e.g. parsley, basil or coriander

1. Grill the pepper halves until blackened. Place in a bowl and cover with clingfilm. Once cold peel off the skins and dice.
2. Heat the oil in a pan and add the chilli, peppers, tomatoes. Stir for a minute then add the sundried tomato paste and vegetable stock. Bring to the boil and simmer for 15 minutes.
3. Place the tofu with the soup in a food processor or liquidizer and liquidize until smooth and creamy. Return to the pan and heat through. Sprinkle over the herbs just before serving.

www.ingramcontent.com/pod-product-compliance
Lightning Source LLC
Chambersburg PA
CBHW071440070526
44578CB00001B/167